FROM MARRIAGE VOWS TO GOLDEN YEARS

From Marriage Vows to Golden Years

A simple guide to navigating the ups and downs of marriage and building a joyful partnership

Amar Ochani

From Marriage Vows to Golden Years
Copyright © 2025 by Amar Ochani

All rights reserved. No part of this publication may be reproduced, distributed, or transmitted in any form or by any means, including photocopying, recording, or other electronic or mechanical methods, without the prior written permission of the author, except in the case of brief quotations embodied in critical reviews and certain other non-commercial uses permitted by copyright law.

For more information, including translation and foreign rights, please contact the author at amarochani@gmail.com

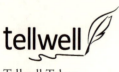

Tellwell Talent
www.tellwell.ca

ISBN
978-1-7750775-4-1 (Paperback)
978-1-7750775-5-8 (eBook)

For Komal

Table of Contents

Author's Note xi
Introduction xiii

"I Do" – The Beginning 1

Building Blocks of a Successful Marriage 3

Mutual Respect 3
Honesty and Trust 4
Communication and Discussion 6
Transparency and Vulnerability 8
Commitment 9
Acknowledgement and Appreciation 10
Companionship 11
Believing in Each Other 12
Sensitivity 13
Sex and Intimacy 13
Learning to Let Go 14
Self-Restraint 15
Assertiveness 16
Shared Vision 17
Common Interests 20
Genuine Consensus 20
Financial Independence 21
Individuality and Interdependence 21
Cooperation and Mutual Learning 22
Children and Family 23

Division of Responsibilities 24
Team Spirit 25
Family Is Our Mirror 26
Home Is Where the Heart Is 27
Parental Support 28
Being Understood 29
Love 32

What Undermines a Marriage 36

Frequent Arguments 36
Silent Treatment 37
Lack of Tolerance 38
Lack of Unity 38
Different Parenting Styles 39
Lack of Thoughtfulness 40
Loss of Interest 41
Uncontrolled Anger 42
Diverse Family Backgrounds 43
Misplaced Priorities 44
Constant Complaints 45
Marriage Doubts 46
Lack of a Balanced Approach 47
Unrealistic Expectations 48

Exploring the Six Types of Marriages 49

Ideal Marriage 49
Successful Marriage 50
Practical Marriage 50
Silent Marriage 51
Arranged Marriage 51
Unhappy Marriage 52
What I Know Now 52

Pre-Marriage Phase 54

　Know Your Partner 54
　Shared Values 55
　Complementary Personalities 55
　Common Interests 56
　Cultural Backgrounds 57
　Pre-Marriage Assumptions 57

Divorce: A Last Resort 59

　Looking Ahead 66

Golden Years of Life 69

　Finding Joy in Aging 69
　The Parent–Child Relationship
　　in the Golden Years 76
　Life After Loss of Spouse 78
　Reflections on the Golden Years of Life 81
　Embracing the Joy of Slowing Down 82
　Balancing Financial Freedom
　　and Peace of Mind 83
　Maintaining Health and Well-Being 84
　Embracing Change 85
　Avoiding Stereotypes 85
　Living Lightly 88
　Liberating Power of Embracing Impermanence 89
　Letting Go of Control and Enjoying the
　　Anticipation 90
　Prioritizing Our Partner 91
　Finding Love in Later Years 91
　Discovering Hidden Talents 92
　Spirit of Giving 93

Be a Storyteller 94
Aging Gracefully 95
Staying Relevant in Later Years 96
Making the Most of Our Golden Years 97
Beauty of Solitude 98
Cherishing Memories 98
Embracing Self-Acceptance 99
Embracing Imperfection 100
Kindness Always Matters 101
Navigating Life's Surprises 102
A Life Well-Lived 103
What I Know Now 104

Afterword 105
Life Principles 109
Acknowledgements 111

Author's Note

When I decided to take a break from regularly sharing my thoughts and essays in November 2022, little did I know I would start working on my second book within a month. The inspiration was our forthcoming golden jubilee anniversary in December.

One day, as I visualized how the family would celebrate, I thought, "What if my grandchildren asked me to share my experience of fifty years of married life? What would I share?" After several attempts to answer the question, I asked myself, "Why don't I write and present a book on the secret of success in marriage to my wife and family?

Initially, I had some misgivings about venturing into new territory. (My first book was a collection of my motivational thoughts and essays.) However, looking retrospectively, I was sold on writing a book on the secret of a successful marriage. *It was an idea whose time had come.*

> It was dinner time, a few days after the family had celebrated our Golden Jubilee Anniversary in a heartwarming

way—which has become and will always remain etched in our memories—when I said to my family members, "Let's share our New Year's resolutions."

Each one of us began sharing our goals for 2023. When my turn came, I did not have any doubt whatsoever about what my New Year's resolution would be. I said, "I will write a book." With that declaration, the idea became a reality.

It's said that when an idea whose time has come gains momentum, it attracts other ideas to unfold one by one, moving forward in unison. That's how a book conceived as an offering to share the secrets of a successful marriage came to include the topics of Pre-Marriage, Divorce, and Golden Years and became a simple, all-inclusive guide for anyone looking for a real-life narrative on life's journey.

Introduction

Every phase of life offers opportunities and challenges. How best we use the opportunities and face the challenges determines the quality of our relationships and degree of success in achieving our goals, whether we are preparing to get married, looking to make our married life more meaningful and satisfying, or seeking to enjoy a peaceful and fulfilling retirement.

This book is based on the conviction that although life doesn't always go according to plan, we can be better prepared to handle challenges and make the most of opportunities if we thoughtfully set our priorities and dedicate time and effort to learning the necessary skills and developing the required characteristics for success in marriage.

For example, if we are preparing to get married, we must consider whether the person we will spend our life with meets our aspirations of an ideal partner. How do I get to know my potential partner well enough to make life's most important decision? How do I create a joyous, meaningful, and long-lasting relationship with my partner? Do I have the skills necessary to handle the ups and downs of married life? If not, how do I learn them? How do I raise a loving family that roots for each other and contributes towards the creation of a harmonious and supportive space?

There are times when despite our best intentions, things don't work out. How do we handle such situations with grace and empathy?

The golden years are a time to relax and enjoy life's closing chapter. They're also an opportunity to infuse it with purpose and leave behind lasting memories. How do we let go of control and make peace with changed roles where we are no longer in the driver's seat? How does the practice of gratitude and forgiveness affect our experience in later years?

From Marriage Vows to Golden Years attempts to answer the above questions and provides practical guidelines we can apply in our daily lives. I share these lessons from the perspective of someone who has seen these dynamics play out in real-life situations and who has made a fair share of mistakes. I learned from first-hand experience what works and what doesn't work in relationships.

Fifty-two years ago, I married Komal in a traditional, Indian way. It has been a fascinating journey, from entering into marriage as total strangers to today, where I can't think of life without Komal. In the Afterword, she beautifully summarizes our long journey and shares the secret of our successful marriage despite our different outlooks.

When I married, I was an angry young man who thought the world of himself—not that I realized it then. I controlled my temper very nicely when dealing with outside people, but when it came to interacting with my family, mainly Komal, all restraints fell apart. I did have redeeming features. I loved my family—I still do—and I had a humanitarian streak in me; I can't hold the grudge for a long time.

Has marriage changed me through the years? You bet. There is so much one can learn from a partner. Komal has been my best resource for confronting my limitations and cultivating patience and tolerance. Both partners, indeed, need to work on the marriage. One must also work on oneself to improve the chances of marital success. Embracing personal growth has a ripple effect on those around us.

Sometimes, it's natural to be anxious or overwhelmed with the state of our marriage and wonder where we are headed. *From Marriage Vows to Golden Years* aims to inspire readers to create new possibilities for their relationships. I hope to encourage you to implement suggestions and follow the guidelines (based on my fifty-two years' lived experience and the lessons drawn from observing other couples) that can positively impact your marriage, and help you build a more meaningful and satisfying relationship.

We, or the conditions we live in, will never be perfect. Mistakes are inevitable. By the time we have learned lessons from our past mistakes, we are ready to make new ones. We must continue adapting, learning, and adjusting to find common ground. Relationships don't thrive by default, and marriage and family are no exception. They need to be nurtured on an ongoing basis.

I hope this book is a helpful resource in every stage of your life.

"I Do" – The Beginning

Marriage is a beautiful union of two people who come together to start a new life as one. It holds the promise of creating a future in which their individual dreams merge to become more significant than they could ever be alone. It's a win–win situation like no other, and it's beautiful to see two people truly and deeply in love.

Marriage is not a matter of convenience but a commitment to stay loyal and supportive of each other through thick and thin.

Finding one's soulmate is indeed a stroke of good fortune, and making a lifelong commitment to that person is something to be proud of. Commitment takes work and effort, and not everyone is willing to do that. Overcoming the natural resistance to commitment is a sign of strength and dedication and it sets you apart from those who doubt the power of true love.

However, marriage is not a fairy tale. It does not succeed by chance or fate. It requires constant effort and dedication from both partners to make it work. No marriage is perfect because we who make the marriage are imperfect. We have flaws, weaknesses, and disagreements that can challenge our relationship.

But these challenges are also opportunities to grow and learn from each other.

The success of marriage comes from laying the building blocks of its edifice one by one. It comes from respecting each other's differences, communicating honestly and openly, compromising when needed, forgiving when hurt, and celebrating when happy. It comes from nurturing the love that brought them together in the first place and keeping it alive and fresh throughout the years.

Marriage is a gift that we give to ourselves and our partners. It is a way of expressing our deepest feelings and sharing our most intimate thoughts. It is a blessing that enriches our lives and makes us better people.

Marriage is what we make it. Whether or not marriages are made in the heavens, they succeed or fail mainly for the reasons created on earth. It is up to us to make our marriage a paradise on earth.

Marriage is the triumph of faith over cynicism. Just imagine two people coming together and taking vows to remain faithful to each other for the rest of life. We know that not everyone keeps their vows, but the very act of taking such vows sounds audacious. How do we, then, navigate marriage so that there is a better chance of honouring these vows than breaking them?

Let's explore.

Building Blocks of a Successful Marriage

Mutual Respect

Mutual respect is the foundation of any healthy relationship. If we want to build a successful marriage, this is an essential quality because the consequences of the lack of respect in marriage are far-reaching.

When there is mutual respect in the marriage, partners acknowledge each other's contributions, opinions, and roles. It involves listening and being present to each other. This also means sharing our interests, passions, dreams, and fears and supporting each other in their goals and challenges.

We all make mistakes, but one thing we should never do is intentionally hurt our partners. Mutual respect is about accepting each other for who we are and making a conscious effort to treat one another with kindness, even when things get tough. Gentleness melts away hard feelings and gives rise to respect and love.

No amount of external factors, such as money, success, social standing, or even attempts to patch up a relationship, can compensate for a lack of respect. On the other hand, when partners work to build respect in the relationship, they ensure that their marriage is on firm footing and they are on the road to a successful and enriching partnership.

"Every good relationship, especially marriage, is based on respect. If it is not based on respect, nothing that appears to be good will last very long." —Amy Grant

Priyanka Chopra, an Indian actress and singer, once shared her thoughts on the importance of mutual respect in a relationship. In an interview with *PEOPLE*, reported by www.lovebscott.com, she said, "He has to be someone who respects you. Then everything is so easy because you give each other credit for your intelligence, you give each other the benefit of the doubt because you trust each other. There is so much that comes out of that."

Honesty and Trust

Honesty and trust build confidence and security in the marriage. Honesty between partners is more than being faithful to each other. We must express ourselves truthfully with each other and be willing to be open and vulnerable. Honesty represents our commitment to a lifelong relationship. Honesty creates trust and intimacy among partners.

Trust is the cornerstone of a marriage. Without it, the relationship will be shallow and superficial, no matter how long it continues. Trust allows partners to be comfortable with each other. They are more likely to forgive and give the benefit of the doubt when they trust each other. It also helps in building consensus and it is a healthy mechanism for resolving differences that are bound to crop in any honest relationship. Trust is a declaration partners give to one another, saying, "You can count on me."

"The best proof of love is trust." —Joyce Brother

Trust comes when partners give space to each other to express themselves openly. Every time a partner listens with empathy and is present to their partner, the space for expression expands. Conversely, if a partner shows impatience or, worse, is angry, the space shrinks. With repeat scenarios, a pattern is set, and they either come closer and radiate warmth or become distant and go into their little shells. When there is trust, couples can work together to overcome obstacles and keep their love alive and well. Without it, however, even the strongest bond can quickly deteriorate.

It's about having faith in each other's intentions and abilities and trusting each other to make the best decisions for themselves and their relationship, which can lead to a productive and empowering partnership.

Keeping our promises, retracing our steps, apologizing when we are wrong, and responsibly clarifying doubts with our partner goes a long way in building mutual trust.

Communication and Discussion

Communication is the lifeline of marriage. Unfortunately, many marriages lose their spark and passion due to a lack of communication. Disagreements and arguments are normal in any relationship, including marriage. The key is to handle them with care and thoughtfulness, be mindful of our words, and choose them carefully, especially during heated conversations. Even in the midst of a disagreement, we can still be respectful and kind to our partners. There is always a gentle way to express our thoughts and feelings.

When communication breaks down, it can create distance and make it difficult to have heart-to-heart conversations. So, it is worthwhile to make an effort to keep the lines of communication open and to stay connected with the partner. If something about our partner bothers us, we must convey it clearly without blame or guilt. Communication is a tool to share our needs and expectations with our partners. We can't expect our partners to read our minds.

"Good communication is the lifeblood of a successful marriage, so when spouses stop talking

at deep level, their marriages slowly begin to die. After all, a marriage will only be as good as a couple's communication." —Dr. Greg Smalley

Couples can set some ground rules to resolve conflicts and repair strained relationships. These rules should be transparent and fair to both partners.

For example, one such rule could be never letting a prolonged silence linger for too long after an argument or disagreement. When our minds are left to their own devices, they can amplify negativity and create justifications for our actions or words. Engaging in conversation with your partner, even if it's just a few sentences, can prevent negativity from festering and get the situation back to normal.

It's natural to resist bringing up something uncomfortable to talk about. However, let's consider that avoiding tough conversations leads to further issues down the line and can create assumptions and misunderstandings. Remember: Engagement, not avoidance, can help create an open, honest dialogue between partners.

Effective communication is a two-way process that involves both speaking and listening. When one person is speaking, the other person must be attentive and actively listen to what is being said. Likewise, when the other person speaks, the roles must reverse, and the first person must listen. This way, both parties can understand each other's point of view and have a productive conversation.

"The first duty of love is to listen." —*Paul Tillich*

Communication is necessary in any situation, such as when we share our joys and sorrows and our hopes and fears with our loved ones, not just when conflicts arise or during serious talks. Small talk is just as important as deep and meaningful conversations. Sharing everyday experiences can warm our relationship, bring us closer, and help us feel more connected.

Transparency and Vulnerability

Since we are discussing the importance of open communication in a relationship, I must also emphasize the value of transparency and vulnerability.

Transparency builds trust between partners and requires being truthful and open about our thoughts and emotions. For instance, if you feel lonely at home while your partner is out enjoying long walks, share your feelings with them. Similarly, if one believes their partner disregards their input or takes it for granted, it helps to clear the clouds by speaking out and matter-of-factly expressing one's thoughts without blaming or feeling guilty.

By being honest about your fears, likes, and dislikes without trying to present a false front, you enable your partner to understand where you stand and give them a chance to do something about it.

> *"Transparency is the foundation of communication."* —Steve Maraboli

Vulnerability creates a deeper connection with a partner. It involves taking risks and letting your partner see your authentic self, including your innermost thoughts and feelings. After all, who better to share these with than your soulmate?

A relationship can stagnate if one or both of the partners are always on guard, constantly trying to avoid upsetting the other. For example, if one partner struggles to keep up with the other's hectic lifestyle but is afraid to express their feelings for fear of upsetting the balance, the relationship may lack depth.

You are taking a risk by being vulnerable and sharing your emotions with your partner. Agreed. But the rewards are worth the risk, including a more profound connection, greater understanding, and a satisfying relationship. These situations offer opportunities to go beyond surface-level interactions and make our marriages more meaningful and fulfilling.

> *"Vulnerability is the only bridge to build connection."* —Brene Brown

Commitment

While likes and dislikes may change, a commitment can help partners stay the course even when faced with obstacles and challenges. It brings them closer and builds trust and loyalty.

Commitment in marriage is not just about living together; it's an unwavering promise to support each other through life's journey. Commitment means choosing your partner again and again, in both the good times and bad, and it's this choice that forms the bedrock of an enduring marriage.

Acknowledgement and Appreciation

Marriages flourish when couples practice appreciation and acknowledgement in their daily lives. It keeps the relationship between partners fresh and alive. When partners acknowledge each other's efforts and contributions, they feel valued and appreciated, which brings them closer and strengthens their connection. Conversely, a lack of acknowledgement and appreciation keeps a marriage subdued and prevents it from blossoming. Lack of acknowledgement blocks out spontaneity and generosity in a relationship.

The small things count, and showing genuine appreciation for what your partner has done or said can brighten their day. And we don't have to wait for an occasion; simply having them in our life is a gift worth acknowledging.

So, take time to acknowledge your partner and all they do, and watch as your love and respect for each other deepen and grow.

*"Acknowledgement is the only way to
keep love alive." —Barry Long*

Companionship

*"The best thing to hold onto in life is
each other" —Audrey Hepburn*

Companionship is the juice of a relationship. When two people create a special place for each other in their hearts, it makes the marriage feel magical. It's important to constantly nurture and cherish this companionship to keep the love and connection alive.

Over time, we get set in our ways, and changing how we relate and interact with each other becomes quite challenging. However, if we were to sit back and introspect a little, it would become clear to us that it's worthwhile to go through a bit of awkwardness to relate newly to our partner.

Spending time with our partner is something we should look forward to, just as we do with our close friends. Whether going on a date night, taking a vacation, or spending an evening at home, dedicating time to one another can help maintain a robust and healthy relationship. Although socializing and participating in community events makes life exciting and gives us visibility, being comfortable and content with each other's company builds confidence in marriage, and the partners feel reassured.

If we find ourselves regularly seeking the company of others to enjoy our leisure time, it may be a sign that something is missing in our relationship. It takes effort to discover new things about our partner and our relationship, but it keeps the spark alive. And it's not as hard as it might sound. The trick is to learn to share our thoughts and feelings with our partners.

I am not very talkative or effusive by nature. But I have learned to make small talk, say funny things that sometimes sound silly, and try to brighten up the situation when I see Komal is not in a good mood or is a bit gloomy. My favourite one is starting to sing a Bollywood song or saying how beautiful she looks. It never fails.

Believing in Each Other

When we have faith in our partner, we don't feel the need to argue or question each other's decisions because we know our partner will always act with integrity and consideration towards us and always have our best interests at heart. We have inner confidence in our partners that they will be appropriate in their deeds and words. They will act respectfully in the presence of friends, family, and the public. We are relaxed and exude a sense of assurance and quiet confidence.

Also, we are not afraid to express different viewpoints or opinions because we are confident that our partner will listen and understand.

Sensitivity

Marriage is like building a beautiful house brick by brick, except that the building blocks of a successful marriage are invisible. Still, their presence is undeniable in the households filled with joy and happiness.

Sensitivity is an excellent quality that comes from having a beautiful heart. A sensitive person is someone who can feel the pain of another person and will avoid using harsh words when communicating with others. They intuitively know when it is time to speak up and when it's time to listen.

However, a relationship should not be so fragile that it can't handle disagreements and differences of opinion. It's natural for partners to have differing viewpoints, and it's a mark of maturity to resolve such differences with respect and understanding without putting the other partner on the defensive.

Sex and Intimacy

Sex enhances intimacy and connection between partners. However, sex alone cannot sustain a relationship. Bodies happily come together when the minds and hearts are united.

Therefore, sex should be seen as an expression of love and affection, not as an obligation or a reward. Partners should communicate their needs and desires openly and respectfully and be attentive to each other's signals and cues. They should also be willing to experiment and spice things up occasionally to keep the spark alive.

April Eldemire, a licensed marriage and family therapist, emphasizes both physical and emotional intimacy, and in a *Psychology Today* article, says, "I encourage couples to think about physical and emotional intimacy as components that work in tandem with each other to create a healthy and fit relationship. Improving the strength of both will improve and balance out the health of your relationship overall."

Learning to Let Go

Letting go is not just a one-time act; it is a way of life. In marriage, it's an indispensable tool to avoid getting stuck. No one is perfect. Sometimes, we say or do things that upset our partners, and vice versa. That is why learning to let go, besides being compassionate, makes practical sense. Holding onto trivial issues will only cause unnecessary stress and arguments. So, let's learn to let go and enjoy a more peaceful and fulfilling life.

"Holding on is believing that there's only a past; letting go is believing that there's a future." —Daphne Rose Kingma

William Hwang, Psy. D., a licensed clinical psychologist, shared the benefits of relinquishing our frustrations in an article for *Psychology Today*. He says, "Letting go allows us to channel our mental, emotional, and physical energy in a productive way. It is the psychological equivalent of flipping a switch from a focus on how things 'should' have gone a certain way to a focus on what we can do now."

Self-Restraint

Self-restraint helps us avoid unnecessary conflicts and maintain a healthy dynamic with our partners by controlling our impulses and emotions. Both partners must work together to develop self-restraint, as it can prevent one person's negative behaviour from escalating and causing irreparable harm to the relationship.

For example, in the heat of an argument, it can be tempting to say things that we really don't mean. Self-restraint can help us avoid saying something hurtful we might regret later.

Practicing self-restraint can instill patience and resilience. It allows couples to deal with minor irritants or major challenges with grace and compassion, and promote a healthier and more respectful relationship.

It's about choosing the right moment and the right words that can make all the difference.

Assertiveness

Marriage is a journey that requires partners to think as a couple, as a family. Differences in opinions, tastes, likes and dislikes, expectations, and parenting ideas that remain dormant in the first flush of marital bliss begin to surface with time. Compromise, adjustment, and give-and-take are indispensable tools for managing married life and making it successful.

Unfortunately, unexpected challenges may test the patience and assumptions of partners. Sometimes, asserting our feelings and letting our partner know what we are missing is necessary for marriage success. Appeasement never pays off in the long run, and practicing assertiveness calmly and respectfully whenever required helps to clear the clouds.

Being assertive doesn't mean being aggressive or harsh. It's about communicating our needs or feelings honestly and respectfully to our partner to remove irritants from the relationship and create a win–win situation. We tend to shy away from expressing ourselves directly. However, when practiced with empathy and commitment to strengthen a relationship, assertiveness brings partners closer and deepens their mutual respect and trust.

Shared Vision

The importance of shared vision in marriage can hardly be over-emphasized. A shared vision helps partners set goals and realize their dreams. It creates a bond of unity that gives meaning and purpose to marriage.

An empowering family vision includes creating a loving, nurturing, and safe space in which all members care for each other and are committed to supporting one another in their physical, mental, and emotional development with respect and appreciation for each other's contribution.

By sharing their vision, family members can make it more real and inspire one another to achieve their goals. For example, family members can share their thoughts over a dinner. Or they can have family meetings from time to time to exchange their views, gain clarity, and support each other in facing challenges and create new possibilities.

"A shared vision with shared values and good communication where both spouses take positive action can make a beautiful marriage." —Marnie Kuhns

Sometimes, a message given at a critical time can create a vision that becomes the driving force for the rest of life.

I lived with my family in London, England, for four years to complete my banking assignment. I left London in April 1993 to report back to my employers in India.

On the advice of our friends, we, as a family, decided to leave our two sons, aged sixteen and seventeen behind in London to pursue their studies. My wife would remain in London to make necessary arrangements for the children then join me after a few months.

While writing this chapter, I asked Komal whether she would like to share how it was for her going through that demanding time. The following are her reminiscences:

> In mid-1993, we had to return to India from London. We wanted to settle our sixteen- and seventeen-year-old boys so they could pursue their studies in London. Amar had to leave for India immediately, as his tenure in the UK had expired, and we needed to get our daughter, who was ten years old, admitted to a good school in India. I stayed back with the boys.
>
> It was a perfect time to spend two months with the boys to understand them and help them understand the situation. We three bonded well. I was not at ease thinking about how these teenagers would manage alone, what they would do, etc. It was necessary to tell the children about moral values and the realities of life.

Every day, we talked about one issue or another. They listened and talked as well. We rented a room for them in a shared apartment. They prepared themselves to work part-time to pay for their living expenses. They started working before I left.

I used to cook their favourite food daily, have loving talks and encouraging conversation, and the time came when I had to leave. It was time to sit with the children and leave them with a few lessons:

They must look after each other.

We are service people from middle-class families. If they study well, they can progress and live a good life.

They must keep good company, live honestly and truthfully, and not even look at the things that don't belong to them. If their conduct is upright and straight, they will be happy.

The vision shared between mother and sons in those two crucial months was life-changing for the boys and has shaped their lives.

Common Interests

Common interests keep the relationship exciting and fun. It enhances the marriage if partners can appreciate and enjoy a few activities or hobbies together. And it's not so hard to pick up a couple of partner's interests and enjoy them together. It's about balancing mutual interests and respecting each other's preferences.

Having common interests can bring partners closer and warm their relationship. All we need is a little thoughtfulness and mutual understanding.

Genuine Consensus

"If you want to go quickly, go alone. If you want to go far, go together." —African proverb

Genuine consensus solidifies the partnership, and makes it possible for couples to work together to build their small world where everyone feels heard. It also takes listening patiently to your partner's point of view, and working through differences to bridge the gap.

When both partners are actively involved in making decisions and are interested in each other's opinions and inputs, they bring out the best in each other and make the family a more effective and productive unit.

Financial Independence

Financial independence gives confidence and peace of mind. Money is not everything, but we need enough to live comfortably and plan for our family's future. Financial security is also required to face life's uncertainties.

Having sufficient income to satisfy our needs and the needs of those who depend on us is a great morale booster and makes it possible to plan our activities with certainty. Whether entertaining friends, planning holidays, saving for the education of our children, or building a retirement nest, all this is possible when we have sufficient income resources.

At the same time, it's also necessary to prudently manage our expenses and live within our means, Calvin Coolidge, thirtieth President of United States, once said, "There is no dignity quite so impressive, and no independence quite so important, as living within your means."

Individuality and Interdependence

Interdependence in marriage is often misunderstood and seen as a weakness, but in reality, it's a strength. Celebrating and embracing the interdependence between two partners creates a balance in a relationship. By working together, the partners can better understand one another's strengths and weaknesses. Then, they can rely on one another to contribute their best efforts to manage their household and achieve long-term goals more effectively.

For example, one partner may be good at entertaining children and encouraging them to shine in sports and outdoor activities. The other partner may be good at helping children to excel in academics. Both can contribute their skills to bring out the best in their children, and they can appreciate and learn from each other. By balancing individuality and interdependence, they can achieve great things as a family. Dr. Stephen Covey, the author of *The 7 Habits of Highly Effective People*, says, "Independent people combine their own efforts with the efforts of others to achieve their greatest success."

Cooperation and Mutual Learning

In a marriage, cooperation is more important than competition. When two people marry, they do so to build a life together and support each other's dreams and goals. While some healthy competition can be motivating and fun, it should never come at the expense of cooperation and working together towards common objectives. The beauty of marriage is that both partners bring their unique experiences and perspectives to the table, making it mutually beneficial to learn from one another. By welcoming the spirit of cooperation and mutual learning, couples can continue to grow, shine, and enjoy shared accomplishments.

> *"Marriage, in its truest sense, is a partnership of equals, with neither exercising dominion over the other, but, rather, with each encouraging and assisting the other in whatever responsibilities and aspirations he or she might have." —Gordon B. Hinckley*

Children and Family

Children give us new purpose and motivation to succeed and excel in life. They motivate us to be our best selves, not just for own success, but also to set an example and provide for them. It's a beautiful cycle of inspiration that continues with each generation. (I would like to acknowledge that many highly accomplished couples don't have children for various reasons.)

However, the marital relationship is the primary relationship in the marriage. Sometimes, we tend to neglect it and go overboard as we focus on children.

A rule that can go a long way in eliminating or reducing friction between the partners is to avoid sitting in judgement on disputes and disagreements between kids and spouse. A better way is to encourage children to settle disputes with the concerned spouse.

When parents work together and support each other in raising children, it creates a positive and nurturing environment where children can grow and thrive and are on the path to a successful future.

"I think that enduring, committed love between a married couple, along with raising children, is the most noble act anyone can aspire to." —Nicholas Sparks

Division of Responsibilities

Running a household is a joint responsibility of husband and wife, and children can join in when they reach adulthood.

Understanding each one's responsibility is necessary for efficient household running. However, we must communicate our preferences, choices, likes, and dislikes to each other on ongoing issues. Home is a dynamic entity. We can't set boundaries for once and for all and say, *Now it's your problem*. It is good to have mutual discussions about buying anything new, such as furniture, appliances, and interior changes. It not only makes for a better decision but also gives everyone in the family a feeling of participation.

For instance, buying a new sofa can be an occasion to sit together and discuss budget, colour, size, and style. Similarly, discussing the layout, materials, and timeline when buying or renovating the kitchen will allow everyone in the family to provide input and feel involved in decision-making. When planning a family vacation, agree on the destination, duration, and activities everyone will enjoy. This way, everyone's opinions and preferences are considered, leading to a happier and more harmonious household.

In 2005, we moved from a rental accommodation in Surrey, BC, to our own condo in Coquitlam, BC. It was an exciting but testing experience to furnish the apartment within a limited budget and timeframe. Three of us, my wife, my daughter, and I, would head off in the morning, visit stores like Ikea, Hudson's Bay, or Bombay Company, and return tired in the evening. Soon, we realized that if we were to complete our task satisfactorily, we must agree on some rules, as otherwise, we would be wasting our time trying to convince one another of our preferences. So, the rule we agreed upon was that we would purchase an item only when we all agreed. It was like a turnaround. Each of us realized that we must give and take. If I need to buy a dining table of my choice, I must agree to buy a sofa of my daughter's choice, a bedroom set of my wife's choice, and so forth. Everything seamlessly fell into place. We could furnish our place within our budget and timeframe, then move in.

Team Spirit

One of the keys to a successful marriage is the family doing things together as a way of life. Eating meals together, going for walks together, and attending parent–teacher meetings together whenever possible are just a few examples of how family can strengthen their bond. Also, discussing and making decisions together makes everyone feel involved.

Conversely, if we don't make a conscious effort to spend time together, it's hard to create a bond that gives everyone in the family a sense of togetherness. It is incredible how much these little things add up and create a true team spirit in the household and lasting memories with loved ones.

"The greatest marriages are built on team work. A mutual respect, a healthy dose of admiration, and a never-ending portion of love and grace." —Fawn Weaver

Family Is Our Mirror

Being with family is a beautiful experience, allowing us to be authentic without any façade.

To be a great partner, parent, or sibling, we must first be good human beings. This entails being truthful, dependable, and compassionate. The family space can be a powerful catalyst for self-improvement, as it mirrors our true selves.

Focusing on our personal growth can help us support each other, creating an empowering home environment. The family unit offers an incredible opportunity for personal development since we won't find a better reflection elsewhere.

There may be times when we may not like what we see in the mirror and say, "This is the wrong mirror," and remain in denial. But we could say, "What I see is not pretty, but a mirror can't lie," and begin the work of self-improvement in earnest.

When can I expect to say my mirror job is done? Truth is, never.

In my fifty-two years of marriage experience, the lesson I have learned most is that there will not come a time when we can say we don't have to work on our marriage anymore. But that's the beauty of it. Learning in marriage, just like in life, never stops.

> *"Family is always a mirror. You can hide from other people, you can even hide from yourself, but your family is going to reflect what you're doing right back at you." —Martina Boone, Illusion*

Home Is Where the Heart Is

There is nothing quite like coming home after a long day. Home is where the heart is, and one always feels comfortable and at ease in one's own space. Whether cooking dinner, snuggled up on the couch with a good book, or just relaxing in bed, there's nothing like the sweet feeling of being at home. As Jane Austin has said, "Ah! There is nothing like staying home for real comfort."

I love the space where I meditate and the corner where I do my creative work. My most enjoyable moments are when I am at leisure, sitting on the chaise near the window overlooking Mt. Baker on a clear day, sipping my morning tea and talking to Komal.

It's true, but the home, however cozy and comfortable, will lack warmth if there is no peace. The home doesn't feel the same on the day Komal and I are in conflict. Having a peaceful home makes a world of difference to our mindset.

Elizabeth Scott, PhD, a well-known wellness coach, author, and health educator, believes in a harmonious home. In an article for VeryWell Mind, she says, "When looking for ways to manage stress, people often overlook one of the simplest and most effective strategies: Creating a peaceful home. Because most of our days begin and end at home, having a peaceful home as your base can help you launch yourself into the world from a less-stressed place each day."

Parental Support

Marriage creates a new family. However, it's still a part of the family tree. As such, the partners' parents have a role in supporting the newly created unit.

For instance, parents can offer guidance on financial matters, child-rearing or household management. They can provide emotional support, encouragement or comfort, but there should be respect for each other's autonomy and boundaries.

The goals are to help their children successfully start a new life and to be available in case of need without interfering or imposing their views.

However, where couples lack parental support (for various reasons), friends and relatives can help, share their experiences, and provide guidance. Couples can also educate themselves by reading books and accessing community services.

Being Understood

Human beings yearn to be understood and acknowledged for who they are. Being understood is the most reassuring feeling in a marriage. When we feel understood, we are more likely to share our innermost thoughts and emotions with our partner without fear of judgement. We feel protected by the trust that our partner will understand our insecurities and limitations. After all, who doesn't have them?

"The beauty of mutual understanding is that it leads to a shared reality." —Juan Carlos Perez Cortes

Fyodor Dostoevsky, one of the greatest novelists of all time, and his wife, Anna Dostoyevskaya, differed in their interests and views. Yet, they had a very happy and enduring marriage.

In the afterword to her memoir, as quoted on the www.themarginalian.org, Anna reflects on the secret to their successful marriage:

> Throughout my life it has always seemed a kind of mystery to me that my good husband not only loved and respected me as many husbands love and respect their wives, but almost worshipped me, as though I were some special being created just for him. And this was true not only at the beginning of our marriage but through all the remaining years of it, up to his very death. Whereas in reality I was not distinguished for my good looks, nor did I possess talent nor any special intellectual cultivation, and I had no more than a secondary education. And yet, despite all that, I earned the profound respect, almost the adoration of a man so creative and brilliant.
>
> Fyodor Dostoevsky, who reflected so much in so much solitude on the deepest problems of the heart, doubtless prized my non-interference in his spiritual and intellectual life. And therefore, he would sometimes say to me, "You are the only woman who ever understood me!" (That was what he

valued above all.)" He looked on me as a rock on which he felt he could lean, or rather rest, and it won't let you fall, and it gives warmth."

It is this, I believe, which explains the astonishing trust my husband had in me and in all my acts, although nothing I ever did transcended the limits of the ordinary. It was these mutual attitudes which enabled both of us to live in the fourteen years of our married life in the greatest happiness possible for human beings on earth.

Mutual understanding is like the invisible glue that holds a successful marriage together. It's the soul of lasting love.

Kelly Baker, MS, LPS, a licensed therapist, wrote about the importance of understanding your partner and being understood yourself in an article called "How to Get to Know Your Partner Better: 17 Effective Ways." She says, "Partners need to feel understood by each other to feel bonded with each other. They want to feel valued, heard, and seen by their partner. And that, in turn, can enhance the happiness of both partners experience within the marriage."

Love

"Love is that condition in which happiness of another person is essential to your own." —Robert A. Heinlein

Love in marriage is incredible. It's about finding someone who completes you and becoming one with that person. When you decide to marry someone, you create a family with them. It may take some time to adjust to thinking as a unit rather than an individual, but you are no longer alone. You have a partner who is there for you through thick and thin. Together, you can conquer anything that comes your way. It's all about working together and being there for each other, no matter what.

Love is not just about the initial attraction we feel for someone. True and abiding love develops through understanding and appreciating one another's flaws. It's okay to make mistakes and apologize; sometimes, to quarrel and reconcile. It's part of growing up and getting to know each other. The ups and downs in marriage should make the relationship stronger, not weaker. Love is a realization that despite these unavoidable stresses in the marriage from time to time, we are happy to share our lives together rather than separately.

Love is truly the soul of marriage. When you have that special someone in your life, you always want to be close to them. You can't stop thinking about them and will do anything to make them happy. It's a beautiful feeling that can make life a celebration.

Then, why does love lose its shine over time and become a distant memory?

Well, the answer lies in the fact that love requires nurturing. It's like a seed all over the tree - in its leaves, trunk, flowers, and branches. A seed became a tree only because it was nurtured by good soil, water, and sunshine, and someone cared for it. Similarly, love also requires nurturing with trust, care, understanding, honesty, communication, appreciation, empathy, and more. When we neglect to pay attention to these essential elements, we are failing our love. However, when we take the time to create these conditions, we do our part to ensure that our love will continue thriving and fulfilling our marriage.

What does it mean to nurture love?

When we talk about nurturing love, we mean caring for our relationship and investing time and effort to nourish it. It also means being present, listening, and consciously letting our partners know they are in our thoughts. For example, we could call them at least once during the day from work or home to enquire how they are doing, remain in touch with them when we are on the go, share daily challenges and successes, give thoughtful gifts, and let them know how much we appreciate it that they are in our lives. Choose what resonates with you; you will find many more ways to touch your partner's heart. Nurturing love doesn't always have to be profound. It can also be light banter, simple words, fun, and humour.

Reflecting on our marriage, I could have been more diligent in keeping in touch with my wife in my work life. I often got engrossed with my office responsibilities. But I have learned how much difference it makes to remain connected with our partner when we are away. Also, I have learned to appreciate my spouse and bring some humour to make the space lighter. It makes a big difference. I have always been a thoughtful gift-giver. It pays to consider what is appropriate for the occasion and what will brighten up our partner. However, what counts is not what we do but how we are with the partner. Whatever we do, big or small, when it is infused with sincerity and love, is bound to touch our partner's heart.

Dwelling on the past doesn't serve us. Instead, use it as a tool to make the present happy and the future more promising. The practice of forgiveness, adjustment, and compromise helps us erase the regrets and resentments of the past and write a new page in the relationship.

Nurturing love also involves being committed to our partner and prioritizing our relationship above all else.

Deals at Costco often tempted me, mainly when I was alone shopping. Komal used to be unhappy when I succumbed to temptation and brought home the goodies. I would explain to her how good that deal was, compare the prices of other vendors, and to not buy it at this price would be a mistake, and so on.

She would say, "But we don't have enough storage, and we don't need it."

She was right. At one point, I realized it was not worth it. Whenever I see something that ignites my craving now, I ask myself, "What's more important, the deal or Komal's happiness?" After that, it doesn't take much to persuade myself to proceed with the shopping list.

This is a very small example, but replicate it in all facets of the relationship and you have a measure of what prioritizing your relationship above all else means. Cherish the love that binds you together in this beautiful journey of life because what nurtures love nurtures marriage.

"Every heart sings a song, incomplete, until another heart whispers back. Those who wish to sing always find a song. At touch of lover, everyone becomes a poet." —Plato

What Undermines a Marriage

When discussing what undermines a marriage, we're not referring to the complete breakdown of the relationship. Instead, we're looking at the factors that erode marital harmony and subtly create distance between partners over time. If not dealt with carefully and earnestly in a timely manner, they can create barriers between partners and prevent them from building a joyful partnership.

Frequent Arguments

"Arguing isn't communication, it's noise." —Tony Gaskins

Arguments can set partners on a collision course. When two people engage in a heated debate, it can create a win–lose situation where one person comes out on top while the other feels defeated. This dynamic is unhealthy for a relationship, as it can lead to resentment, mistrust, and distance between partners. Couples need to work through disagreements respectfully and productively.

Silent Treatment

"Silence is argument carried out by other means." —Che Guevara

Silence is a powerful tool in any relationship. When a relationship is founded on trust, partners can find comfort in silence without feeling uneasy. However, silence can also be a dangerous weapon when used to hurt or settle scores between partners or to manipulate and control the other person. In these cases, silence can become a deadly form of treatment that can cause more harm than words ever could.

Sheri Stritof, author and marriage consultant, in her article "Impact of Silent Treatment in Relationships," says, "When silence, or, rather, the refusal to engage in a conversation, is used as a control tactic to exert power in a relationship, then it becomes 'the silent treatment,' which is toxic, unhealthy, and abusive. But, if being silent means simply taking a timeout to think things through and then address the issue again later, that is not at all the same thing."

Lack of Tolerance

Lack of tolerance constrains our growth as individuals and as a family and undermines the capabilities and talents partners can contribute to each other and the family. We must recognize that no one is perfect, including our partners, but we unfortunately forget this in practice. Understanding their strengths and weaknesses requires genuine acceptance and a willingness to learn and grow together.

Partners can let go of each other's mistakes and lapses when they genuinely accept their imperfections.

"I think we need to develop powerful dose of tolerance to understand each other's humanness. None of us is perfect." —Cathy Burnham Martin

Lack of Unity

"When you make the sacrifice in marriage, you're sacrificing not to each other but to unity in a relationship." —Joseph Campbell

Family matters involve both partners. When one partner makes all the decisions without considering the other's input, it can lead to feelings of exclusion and resentment. This can create a tense and unhappy environment in the household, which could be better for everyone. A happy family is one where both partners feel equally valued and supported.

If left unaddressed for a long time, lack of unity can render a family dysfunctional, as the partners are likely to act on cross-purposes, whether managing the household or making major decisions. The best way is to have an open and honest dialogue to remedy the situation before it takes an emotional toll on partners. Partners can pick a couple of concrete issues and discuss how not taking a united stance has affected the couple and family. That can give us insight into the cost, material and non-material, we are paying by not presenting a united front as a couple and as a family.

Different Parenting Styles

While complementary skills in marriage can be an asset, having entirely different parenting styles can be problematic.

For example, one partner tries to make children think and do things as independently as possible to bring out the best in them and make them self-reliant, while their partner tries to make things easy for their children and often lets them off the hook to show their love and care.

This delicate situation needs to be handled with maturity and forbearance. The parents must realize that it's not about them. The children's future is more important than sticking to their viewpoints. They must be conscious of how their competing ideas affect the children and how this may leave hard feelings between the partners. It may be a good idea to involve children to find out what is working with them and what is not working and modify our approach to facilitate their development. This is possible when both parents are actively involved in the upbringing of their children and there is an ongoing dialogue between them.

Lack of Thoughtfulness

Unnecessary disagreements hurt feelings. They may not lead to conflicts but leave behind avoidable unease.

If we look closely, it will become clear that what spoils the fun in the marriage is mostly trivial—the arguments over petty things and disagreements over issues that are irrelevant to our lives. For example, a partner says," We bought this TV eleven years ago." Another partner disagrees, "No, we bought it twelve years ago." Or, "So and so looks like she is 64 years old." "No, she doesn't look more than 60."

Mindy Carry, a Certified Financial Planner and a life coach, in an article about the arguments most frequently held by couples have over money, has wisely observed, "Each partner must keep in mind that most relationships aren't destroyed by one dramatic act, but series of small acts, even individually inconsequential acts that chip away at your foundation of love and trust."

Correcting your partner over minor mistakes, arguments over things that don't matter much, and little annoyances build up and create distance between the partners rather than bringing them closer. It's prudent to avoid unnecessary disagreements to maintain harmony in marriage. Thoughtfulness works equally inside and outside the household.

Loss of Interest

When couples lose interest in their marriage, it can be a sign that they have been drifting apart for some time without taking action to address the issues. This can undermine the foundation of the relationship and make it difficult to maintain a strong connection. Partners need to share their thoughts and feelings honestly and work together to rekindle their love and commitment to one another.

Here are two scenarios highlighting how addressing this issue proactively and thoughtfully can address this issue effectively.

In the first, Roma and Chris had been married for over a decade. As time passed, they noticed a gradual decline in their emotional connection. The initial excitement had faded, and they found themselves in a routine where they barely communicated beyond daily chores.

Instead of accepting this as a new normal, Roma and Chris decided to rekindle their shared interests. They revisited the activities they used to enjoy together—like hiking, cooking, and dancing. This way, they reignited their passion and discovered new facets of each other. Their renewed enthusiasm brought them closer and they felt more connected than ever.

In the second scenario, Alex and Emily have been married for five years. Emily noticed that Alex was becoming distant, spending more time at work and less time with her. She felt neglected and feared that their marriage was falling apart.

To address it, Emily initiated an honest conversation. She expressed her feelings of loneliness and asked Alex about his perspective. Alex admitted feeling overwhelmed by work stress and personal expectations. Emily encouraged him to share his emotions openly. They attended couples' counselling, where they learned effective communication techniques. By being vulnerable and actively listening to each other, they rebuilt their emotional bond and found ways to support each other.

Each couple's journey is unique, but these stories highlight valuable lessons for maintaining a healthy and connected relationship.

Uncontrolled Anger

Anger is a destructive force in any relationship that can tear people apart. This is especially true in a marriage, where anger can cause partners to distance themselves from each other and harm the overall family dynamic. It can also make it difficult to communicate nicely, and unfortunately, it is often a trigger for domestic violence and abuse.

> *"Anger is an acid that can do more harm to the vessel in which it is stored than to anything on which it poured."* —Mark Twain

Anger is a natural emotion, but how we express and manage it matters. Uncontrolled anger can have a detrimental effect on our physical and mental well-being and our relationships. By exercising self-restraint, practicing introspection, and reflecting on the consequences of anger, we can learn to handle our emotions in a healthy and productive way, leading to a happier and more harmonious life.

Diverse Family Backgrounds

When a couple ties the knot, they bring their individual experiences and family backgrounds, including both of their families. However, things can get tricky if both partners come from different family backgrounds and have different traditions and rules. Both partners need to respect each other's families and not compare them or try to prove that one is better than the other. Instead, couples can work together to bring out the best in both families to create a stronger and more united family unit. This will not only help to bring the partners closer together but also help to build positive relationships between their families.

We cannot deny that the families we grew up in and our parents have influenced our outlook and habits. It's natural to have different upbringings. However, allowing these differences to create disharmony in the family will be unfortunate. While our families will always be a part of our lives, our future is with the family we are starting with our partner, with a new identity, vision, and priorities. It doesn't help to start a new life on a firm footing by pitching our family against our partner's family.

Misplaced Priorities

Family comes first when maintaining a strong and healthy marriage. Competition between partners can weaken the family's foundation. Any differences within the family should be resolved without involving outsiders.

Although social commitments have a place in our lives, they should never take priority over the family's needs. This can be problematic, for example, when one partner is not keen on accepting an invitation from a family friend and the other feels that rejecting it would hurt their feelings. It's always better to discuss such situations calmly and find common ground to avoid misunderstandings or conflicts.

Compromise and adjustment are not signs of weakness, but rather the building blocks of a successful marriage. They greatly help balance different priorities and create a win–win situation. The following example, although hypothetical, captures the spirit of give and take to find common ground.

Jeff and Sophia were newlyweds with a shared dream of owning a house. Jeff envisioned a cozy cottage in the countryside, while Sophia dreamed of a modern apartment in the heart of a city.

They sat down and discussed their priorities. Jeff valued peace and nature, while Sophia craved convenience and social life. They compromised on the location. They found a suburban home with a small garden, close enough to the city for Sophia's work and Jeff's weekend hikes.

Adjustments followed. Sophia agreed to a more rustic interior, and Jeff embraced the idea of a small balcony for Sophia's potted plants. Their dream house became a blend of both their visions—a cozy suburban home with a touch of urban flair. They realized that compromise didn't mean sacrificing their dreams but enriching them through mutual decisions.

Constant Complaints

Complaints squeeze out the joy from married life. It undermines the self-confidence of a spouse constantly targeted by the other spouse. Over time, the situation can become intolerable for the spouse at the receiving end. It's much better to address such concerns as they arise. If the partners communicate their thoughts and feelings frequently, they can avoid flare-ups, and the marital bond can become more resilient as things are not pushed under the carpet. There is ongoing completion.

And, there is a kinder way to express ourselves instead of using harsh words that can only cause harm. Requesting rather than complaining is the best way to communicate your concerns and avoid putting your partner on defence.

> *"Many marriages would be better if the husband and the wife clearly understood that they are on the same side." —Zig Ziglar*

Marriage Doubts

Marriage doubts can be a real challenge and can put a lot of strain on a relationship if they're not dealt with in a right way. One of the biggest factors leading to these doubts is the habit of comparing our relationship to others. Every relationship is unique and should be treated as such.

Doubts in a relationship often arise from a lack of trust and a need for more open communication. Whether it's suspicion of infidelity, financial secrecy, feeling neglected, or resenting your partner's close connections with other people, doubts share these common threads. By recognizing and discussing it calmly, partners feel relieved that they are not alone in their struggles and that they can overcome these issues by opening their hearts to each other.

Suzy Kassem, writer, poet, philosopher, and filmmaker, says, "Doubt kills more dreams than failure ever will." Wise words that underline how doubts can prevent us from reaching our full potential.

Lack of a Balanced Approach

Undoubtedly, the arrival of little ones changes our priorities to some extent. It's natural to love our children. However, sometimes, we tend to focus all our attention and energy on our kids and unintentionally ignore our partners. Our spouse is our life partner and our relationship is the foundation of our family, and a balanced approach can avoid any misunderstandings and help maintain family harmony. The children are delighted to see their parents' love and care for each other.

> *"Happiest families are those in which parents can balance their love for each other with their love for children."* —Bruce Feiler

Unrealistic Expectations

Unrealistic expectations of perpetual passion and a conflict-free married life can set us for disappointment. The initial "honeymoon phase" eventually gives way to a more stable and realistic partnership as couples face day-to-day life with all its vicissitudes. Cultivating candid communication with your partner, working together and setting realistic expectations build resilience and promote a healthy relationship.

Differences and conflicts are normal in any relationship, including marriage. When handled with empathy, understanding, and patience, they can bring partners closer and enhance their mutual respect and trust.

Summing up, it's normal to face challenges in a marriage. By addressing issues that undermine the marriage early on, we can overcome the obstacles that come in the way of creating a fulfilling life with our partner and making our dreams come true.

"I know too many young couples who struggle and think that somehow there's something wrong with them," Michelle Obama, former First Lady of the United States, said during a Good Morning America interview. "And I want them to know that Michelle and Barack Obama, who have a phenomenal marriage and who love each other, we work on our marriage. And we get help with our marriage when we need it."

Exploring the Six Types of Marriages

These marriage types are based on my observation and understanding of marriages around me. As such, the classification has a certain level of arbitrariness. Marriages may have elements of more than one type; marriage dynamics can change over time as a couple gains experience, or unexpected changes in the circumstances may affect partners' behaviour towards each other.

Ideal Marriage

A successful and happy marriage is one where both partners have nurtured their love and cannot imagine their lives without each other. They have overcome obstacles together and have learned to accept each other's flaws. Putting their egos aside for a peaceful and happy family life, they have developed effective ways to resolve conflicts. A marriage based on love is something special that shows in everyday life. The way partners light up in each other's company is inspiring, and it's clear that their marriage is a blessing. There is warmth, understanding, mutual appreciation, and acknowledgment in the relationship. When one partner slips, the other is there to support, not criticize or find faults, which makes a marriage truly remarkable and something to be cherished. It's like what André Maurois, a French author, once said, "A happy marriage is a long conversation which always seems too short."

Successful Marriage

The partners in this marriage have made compromises to find peace and happiness in their family. While they may not consider each other ideal partners, they have developed a mutual respect that allows them to function as an effective team. They recognize that life together is far better than living apart, even if they sometimes feel unfulfilled. The warmth may be missing in the marriage.

> *"Marriage is about compromise; it's about doing something for other person, even when you don't want to." —Nicholas Sparks*

Practical Marriage

For some couples, the well-being of their children is the top priority in their married life. They work together as a team to provide their kids with the best opportunities to thrive academically and in life. They want to save time on personal issues that could distract them from focusing on their children's progress. Their ultimate reward is seeing their children succeed. Although these marriages may not be fulfilling, they can still be successful in their unique way.

Silent Marriage

The fourth type is where the partners have limited engagement. They have their own lives and interests and may not share much with each other. However, they have decided to live together despite their differences. They communicate, when necessary, but they appreciate silence when they are together.

Arranged Marriage

Traditional marriage is a union involving either an arranged or semi-arranged marriage. It is common in Eastern countries. One unique aspect of traditional marriage is that it intertwines married couples' lives with their joint family – a household where multiple generations live together under one roof. This helps families stay close and support each other through the ups and downs of life. This marriage type is declining due to urbanization, population growth, and cultural shifts (changing beliefs, values, and lifestyles) that make living in multi-generational households difficult.

Unhappy Marriage

Lastly, we have a marriage where no love is lost between the partners. It's too late to think of divorce as an option. The marriage is surviving, but it is like a broken car that needs repairs now and then. In some cases, it has been given up and kept as a showpiece as a reminder that it once was a functional car. This type of marriage survives because of cultural influence, religious beliefs, the need to keep up appearances in society, financial considerations, or simply because the couple has resigned themselves to the situation. They're used to being unhappy, and it's their way of life.

What I Know Now

Marriage is not a solo flight. It's a journey of love and commitment that brings two people together to create their small world. Moreover, we can't put marriage on autopilot for long. It's essentially a human endeavour that needs to be cared for and strengthened by both partners.

One can't work on one's marriage without working on oneself. Both go hand-in-hand and sustain each other.

There will always be something that needs to be addressed in marriage. This is a normal part of any relationship. Genuine acceptance of each other's flaws and weaknesses and resolving conflicts respectfully and peacefully is inescapable in a healthy marriage.

Communication is the lifeline of a marriage. It's the only way to share our fears and insecurities, hopes and aspirations, and clear doubts and anxieties. Heart-to-heart conversations reassure both partners that they are not alone and can count on each other. Dialogue lifts the relationship from the surface level, making it complete by bringing warmth and confidence.

Practicing forgiveness and letting go in our daily lives is the best way to prevent grudges from taking root in our hearts and minds.

Unity between the partners makes a family more effective and makes achieving marriage goals possible.

Financial independence and prudent financial management of resources provide stability, a sense of confidence and security, and contribute to peace and harmony in the family.

Finally, being patient and kind to our partner makes a difference—it elevates the relationship from mundane to sublime. With little effort and much love, you can build a joyful and lasting partnership that will stand the test of time.

Pre-Marriage Phase

Laying a Strong Foundation for a Successful Marriage

Before we say "I do," we have the power to shape the future of our marriage. That's why we must take the pre-marriage phase seriously and cultivate the seeds of success as we embark on this new journey. By taking a closer look at what we can do to set ourselves up for a healthy and fulfilling relationship, we can increase the chances of having a happy and enduring marriage.

Know Your Partner

Where do we start when considering marriage? We get to know our partner well. While physical attraction, shared interests, and financial stability matter, we must feel a deep love and respect for a person and be willing to face life's challenges together.

Choose a partner you can trust and believe in, looking beyond surface-level qualities to discover their essence and decide whether they mirror your aspirations and beliefs. With love and support, it's possible to weather the ups and downs of life together, even if your partner experiences setbacks.

Shared Values

When considering marriage, make sure you and your partner share similar values. If your partner is kind, considerate, and open with you, it may be a good sign that you are with the right person. Avoiding excessive materialistic tendencies and secrecy is also important, so look for a partner who values honesty and transparency.

We are or become what our values and beliefs are. If you want to spend your life with a person in marriage, you want to take the time now to understand their values and beliefs, as these genuinely define a person and determine the long-term success of marriage. While there is no harm in considering a person's qualifications and financial status, they should not be the sole basis for choosing a life partner. Consider them, but never compromise your values and what truly matters to you.

Complementary Personalities

Having complementary personalities can be beneficial in a marriage. They can bring different strengths and ideas to marriage. For example, one partner is action-oriented but finds details and planning cumbersome, while the other is detail-oriented and strong in planning. They will complement each other very well and make an excellent team.

However, having a complementary personality is not the only factor contributing to a successful marriage. Other aspects, like, open communication, mutual respect, shared values, understanding, and willingness to work through challenges together, are also required.

Ultimately, what matters most is that both partners feel understood, supported and loved. It's about finding a balance that works for both individuals and allows them to grow together.

Common Interests

Everyone, indeed, has unique tastes and interests. However, it helps if couples have some common interests. For example, if both partners are outdoor enthusiasts, they can spend more time together. Having common interests will add spice to a relationship.

However, having common interests is not a make-it-or-break-it attribute. Other factors, which we have discussed before, contribute to marriage success. So, it may be a good idea to have a dialogue before making up your mind. Besides, it's possible to pick up an interest or two of your partner to add zest to a relationship, provided both people are flexible.

Cultural Backgrounds

When tying the knot, it helps to consider both partners' cultural backgrounds. This doesn't mean that both partners must have identical backgrounds, nor is it suggested that we should approach this angle with prejudice or suspicion. Having an open and honest dialogue about their backgrounds can help partners identify the areas they must work on to achieve mutual understanding, such as beliefs and customs of each other's family.

While having a similar cultural background is helpful, it's not a must for marriage success. Many couples with different cultural backgrounds have also built strong and lasting relationships.

Pre-Marriage Assumptions

Before making any decisions about marriage, have open and honest conversation with your partner about your expectations and goals for the future. Assuming that your partner shares your values or desires without discussing them can lead to disappointments. It's better to take the time to get to know each other's dreams and expectations and make sure that you're both on the same page before deciding to tie the knot. Marriage is a serious commitment, and it has better chances of success when approaching it with clarity and intention.

> *"Making the wrong assumptions causes pain and suffering to everyone."* —*Jennifer Young*

To sum up, when considering marriage, it is important to look for certain qualities in a potential partner. These qualities include caring and thoughtfulness, openness, honesty, and understanding. While complementary skills and common interests can be helpful, focusing on shared values like mutual respect, trust, communication, love, and kindness is more critical. These values will provide a strong foundation for a happy and healthy relationship and help resolve differences when they arise.

The success of a marriage depends on the choices made by the partners before and after the wedding day. It's, therefore, prudent to approach the decision of a life partner with understanding, not emotion alone.

Divorce: A Last Resort

While it's true that many people go through divorce, that doesn't make it any easier for those going through it. Divorce can be a life-changing event for those involved. The process can be easy or difficult, depending on the circumstances and approach. It's up to us to steer this challenging time with compassion and understanding for everyone involved.

Divorce is not something to be ashamed of, but it should not be taken lightly. It's an option of last resort and should only be considered when the difficulties of staying together outweigh the fear of an uncertain future and the pain of going through the divorce process.

Take a step back

Understandably, emotions can run high during a conflict between the partners, but remember that emotions can change over time. When at the point of considering divorce, take a step back and give yourself the space to process your feelings and reflect on the situation. In many cases, the issues that caused the conflict can be resolved with patience and commitment. Putting ego aside and communicating with your partner can help prevent division and breakdowns. By being open and willing to listen to each other, partners can overcome challenges and rebuild strained relationship.

While it is tempting to point fingers and blame our partner, the reality is that our dissatisfaction might stem from within. It's possible that attending to our own needs and well-being may be the key to feeling happier and more content in our relationships and overall life. Taking care of our well-being positively impacts our relationships with others, as we can better provide love, care and support when we are well and happy.

Identify the root cause of relationship issues

Before deciding on divorce, it helps to identify the issues at hand. These issues may relate to finances, emotions, personality clashes, unmet expectations, suspicions of infidelity, lack of quality time together, or differences in parenting styles. Both partners should create a list of their concerns and express them clearly to determine whether these issues are temporary or long-standing. Additionally, both partners should reflect on what led them to consider this decision and assess whether they have effectively communicated their hurts, concerns, and fears with each other.

Couples should not shy away from seeking the help of a good marital therapist to help them identify and address issues that arise before it's too late.

Create a roadmap for reconciliation

If a couple has reached the breaking point, there must be reasons behind it. If they are genuinely committed to resolving their differences and making the reconciliation process successful, they must earnestly address these issues.

More is required than merely agreeing to change, for example, establishing guidelines to measure progress, as otherwise, it will become an uncertain process.

1. Agree to communicate your issues and grievances. Make a list.
2. Be as specific as possible.
3. Continuously update the list, as communication brings clarity.
4. Regularly review the progress, preferably weekly.
5. Spend more time together, go for long walks and weekend trips when possible.
6. Call each other at least once from the office or home to enquire how the day is going.
7. Share daily challenges and accomplishments, and make small talk.
8. Be present to your partner and listen with empathy.

9. Acknowledge progress or lack thereof during the review meetings.
10. Reinforce the commitment to work on the issues.

Saving a marriage requires a sincere effort from both partners. They must be willing to confront the challenges and do whatever it takes to succeed. Sincere communication can help identify the underlying issues that led to the crisis.

The key to a happy marriage lies in your partner's heart. When the ego takes over, it's like being on a ship without a rudder, tossed around by the waves and winds. Staying grounded, communicating openly, and being persistent keeps marriage on course. The partners mustn't get discouraged by temporary setbacks.

Address the issues head-on and take steps to reconnect with your partner. Both partners need to be proactive in this process. Communication is critical, but it's also important to show your partner that you care and appreciate them. Sometimes, a small gesture can make a big difference and bring you closer together. It takes effort from both partners, but with commitment and dedication, a marriage can be saved.

"Reconciliation is the fastest way to change your life." —Mark Hart

Can a couple bounce back from the brink?

Yes, saving a marriage on the brink of collapse is possible. However, both partners must feel they have a stake (emotional bond, shared responsibilities, family support, and so on) in remaining together and be willing to communicate, give and take, forgive each other, and be realistic about their expectations. Once these prerequisites are satisfied, the couple can address the fundamental causes of marital friction. By accepting each other with open eyes and building respect and trust, the couple can usher in a new beginning in their relationship, benefitting themselves and their children, if any.

On the other hand, there are times when the window of opportunity has passed, and it's better to stop pushing and move on. Divorce is a difficult decision, but it may be necessary for both individuals to find happiness in a different way. It's tough to accept, but acknowledging the reality of a failing marriage is the sensible thing to do. It's a difficult choice, but there are times when it could be the best one for everyone concerned.

If the partners choose to part ways, it's humane and beneficial to both partners to approach the situation with kindness and understanding and to remember that everyone is going through their own struggles.

Create a blueprint for life after divorce

Going into divorce without a proper plan is a mistake, and it may leave you feeling stuck with the existing situation, whatever it may be. Remember, if you have chosen divorce, you must have a clear intent to move on and start fresh.

A plan helps you focus on the future instead of dwelling on the past. It can also give you a sense of direction and control over your life, which is often lost during such a difficult time. Whether creating a budget, finding a new job, or pursuing a new interest, having a plan can help you take the necessary steps to rebuild your life after divorce. It may be challenging at first, but having a clear action plan can give you the motivation and confidence you need to move forward with your life.

Show yourself kindness and patience

Going through a divorce can be such a rollercoaster of emotions. It's natural to feel sad, grieve, and experience loss. However, please remember that you don't have to live with those feelings forever. There is life after divorce, and the past doesn't have to define your future. Try not to dwell on what is history and focus on the future instead.

You can find happiness again, but it may come in new and unexpected ways. Instead of trying to recapture joy from the past, try to discover new sources of happiness. And remember the people who love and support you, like your friends, parents, and siblings. They can help you through this difficult time and bring joy to your life in their own ways.

Divorce is profoundly emotional experience, but it can also be an opportunity to know yourself better. A great way to start piecing yourself together is by jotting down things that bring you joy. This could be anything from reading books, listening to music, going for long walks, watching movies, learning new things, and so much more. Be kind to yourself and take things one step at a time.

Accept and move on

Acceptance makes moving on less complicated. The divorce is successful when both partners move on without leaving a trail of bitterness. Both of them need to experience completion without the shadow of a failed marriage following them.

To achieve this, both parties must be generous with each other about the division of assets and custody of children. Access to and opportunities to spend quality time with the children must be liberally conceded to the partner who doesn't have custody. It can only help to continue friendly relations between the divorced partners. Seeking to even out the score or seeking revenge is a bad idea. It doesn't help anyone. Both partners should collaborate to create a co-parenting relationship to benefit any children involved.

When the partners are honest and transparent, mediation is a better way to resolve their issues amicably. This can make the divorce process faster, cheaper, and less stressful for everyone involved.

Prepare for uncomfortable transitions

Forewarned is forearmed, as they say. Life can change drastically after a divorce, not just for the partners involved but for everyone connected through family and friendship. It's necessary to be prepared for these changes, both emotionally and practically. If young children are involved, the situation can be even more challenging.

Every divorce situation is unique. The couple must cooperate and adjust to make the transition as smooth as possible, benefiting their children and themselves. While things will inevitably get easier over time, preparing for the uncomfortable transition helps. By being forewarned, you can better equip yourself to handle the changes that lie ahead.

Looking Ahead

Divorce doesn't necessarily mean the end of a positive relationship between the partners. While the marriage may have failed, the human connection between two people can still be successful with the right approach. By showing compassion and understanding towards each other's limitations, it's possible to move forward positively, even after a divorce. Sometimes, the best decision is to part ways, but doing so with goodwill for one another can ensure that both individuals can thrive in their future endeavors.

Separation or divorce can change a person's perspective on life and relationships. Regardless of the financial outcome, no one truly wins in a divorce. However, if we let go of blame and avoid self-pity and remorse, we can learn lessons that will help us find new meaning in life.

Couples usually do not decide to divorce lightly. They attempt to reconcile before accepting that their differences are irreconcilable and that they will be happier apart. This realization should bring some humility. While we cannot predict the future, both partners must reassess their 'relationship quotient' for now—skills that contribute to the success of a relationship, such as communication and mutual trust. Therefore, the first lesson of divorce can be a healthy dose of humility.

Divorce can provide both parties ample opportunity for self-reflection and personal growth. If we take the time to introspect and examine the experience objectively, we can learn a lot about ourselves.

During the painful divorce process, family, friends, and relatives often become the primary source of support. This highlights the importance of having a good support system.

As the saying goes, "Tough times don't last, but tough people do." Coming out of a divorce can be a confidence booster, especially when both parties have handled the process gracefully and responsibly.

> *"All endings are also beginnings. We just don't know it at the time." —Mitch Albom*

Golden Years of Life

Finding Joy in Aging

Our priorities shift as we move into the later years of life. Retirement becomes a major focus, when we finally can relax and enjoy the fruits of our labour. For many, this means travelling, pursuing hobbies, and spending quality time with loved ones. However, some challenges, like health issues and losing friends and family members, come with age. With the right mindset—staying positive and embracing the changes—and with a strong support system, the golden years can be a period of peace and joy.

The golden years of life are a time to reflect on the journey you have taken and to cherish the constant companion you have in your spouse. You have experienced joy and sadness, and many of us have raised children who now have their own families. As you enter this new chapter, life is still full of potential and new experiences. Take the time to enjoy the simple things and cherish the company of loved ones. These are the memories that will last a lifetime.

Not everyone is in the same situation as they enter retirement. Let's explore some different scenarios and see how we can approach them. I have arranged these categories based on my observation of people I have encountered. The examples of people I give below are composites and not their real names except for the example given under the spiritualists category. These categories are not rigid. (A separate chapter follows covering life after the loss of a spouse.)

Contented

You and your spouse are immersed in the lives of your children and grandchildren. They are your pride and joy. Social media has been an excellent way to stay connected with your family, even when you can't be together. You share pictures of your family and grandchildren on platforms like WhatsApp and Facebook, and it's always so heartwarming to see love and support from friends and family. Whether living in a joint family (multi-generational household) or having a home near your loved ones, you feel truly blessed. You are happy and content with your life.

I have known Kan and Ritu for a long time. In their late seventies, they live with their children and grandchildren in a joint family. Whenever I call Kan and ask him how he is doing, he replies, "I am grateful, God has been very kind. He has given me more than I deserve." Then he narrates how his son and grandchildren are succeeding in their work, studies, and how they are taking care of them. I remember once he shared how his son sometimes comes into his room and gives him a foot massage. Kan and Ritu are a good example of aging with grace and contentment.

Balanced

Life is great even though you are not as involved in your children's lives as you used to be. You still keep in touch with them regularly, though. You and your spouse live independently of your children and you love it. You enjoy your holidays and love going to casinos. You stay in touch with your friends and have a great circle of people around you. Even though you have aged, you still have the zest for a good life.

Sam and Neena are in their early eighties. Sam is popular with friends and takes a keen interest in communal activities but finds time for his grandchildren. On the other hand, Neena is mostly busy with her family. She regularly babysits for her grandchildren and helps them in every possible way. Both love to travel, take cruises regularly, play cards with friends, and enjoy life while helping their children. They have balanced their enjoyment and parental support.

Forgivers

Your golden years have been filled with love and respect for each other despite differences in interests and temperament. You give each other the space to thrive and have learned to accept each other fully. Your friends and family see you as role models for a healthy and happy relationship.

Savati and Raman are a couple as different as night and day. Raman is an early riser, while Savati prefers to catch up on her sleep. Savati is quite talkative, while Raman is a man of few words. Although Raman has a bit of a temper, Savati remains calm and collected. Savati loves cooking and believes everyone enjoys her meals, while Raman sees food as fuel for the body. Additionally, Savati is a newcomer to social media and enjoys answering any question that comes her way, becoming a commentator on various topics.

Despite their contrasting personalities, they manage to make their marriage work. They give each other the space to be themselves, which means both of them can flourish. They don't let their differences drive them apart; they have learned to appreciate each other for who they are. Their marriage may not be perfect, but they weather the ups and downs of life together. As they entered their golden years, they discovered they could see the bigger picture and forgive each other more easily. They still have moments of annoyance, but never let it affect their love for each other.

> *"A happy marriage is the union of two forgivers."* —Ruth Bell Graham

Couples need to see the bigger picture, especially in later years of life. It's like seeing picture-in-picture on a TV—the larger screen represents life, and the smaller screen is marriage in life. It's not worth making a big deal out of minor disagreements, and partners should try to become more forgiving of each other. Even if they still get annoyed with each other, the annoyance shouldn't last long. It feels so much better and helps maintain peace and harmony.

Spiritualists

Both partners share a spiritual or humanitarian inclination and follow the same path. It's a great blessing for their relationship. It has brought a sense of connection and purpose to their lives. It doesn't mean they have isolated themselves from their families or stopped caring about them. Instead, they view family life as one aspect of a broader purpose. They recognize the preciousness of human existence and strive to make the most of every moment before this life's journey ends.

I can't think of a more inspiring example than renowned teacher S. N. Goenka, lovingly known as Goenkaji, from whom I had the good fortune to learn Vipassana meditation. He was instrumental in spreading

Vipassana meditation worldwide, and his wife, Elachi Devi Goenka, assisted him in this mission till last.

In the Short Biography of Goenkaji, published by Vipassana Research Institute, which Goenkaji founded, it states, "Shortly after his marriage to Illachidevi in 1942, the tumultuous period of the Japanese invasion forced Goenkaji and his family to embark on a perilous exodus from Myanmar to India, a journey fraught with tribulation as they traversed dense forests and towering mountains."

Elachi Devi, affectionately known as Mataji (Respected mother), played a significant role in Goenkaji's life and work. Their partnership was a blend of personal dedication and public service.

Passionate

When one partner is more focused on spirituality or giving back to society, and the other is more focused on worldly matters, it can lead to communication gaps. However, when both partners are willing to accept and respect each other's preferences and allow each other space to pursue their interests while also enjoying each other's company, their golden years can still be filled with happiness and love. It's all about finding a healthy balance and learning to appreciate each other's perspectives.

Herman and Rekha are in their late seventies. Herman is a retired civil servant, and Rekha is a former college teacher. They love travelling and outdoor activities. However, Rekha is a devoted spiritualist, whereas Herman has a more worldly bent of mind. He lets Rekha pursue her spiritual path but doesn't get involved with Rekha's spiritual activities. They both share interests in travelling and outdoor activities, and despite different outlooks on more profound aspects of life, they have abiding love, respect, and care for each other. They are an inspiring example of living life to the fullest and growing together as a couple and an individual, following their passion.

Unhappy

It's sad to think about, but some couples can't find a way to work through their issues, even after years of marriage. It's a shame when what should be a time of contentment and peace turns into constant fighting and tension. Eventually, some couples give up and resign themselves to an unhappy marriage. It's a difficult way to live, but for some people, it's the only option they feel they have.

The key to success in any of these or other scenarios is to see what makes you happy. Whether spending time with family, enjoying your hobbies, or following a spiritual or humanitarian path, find what brings you joy and feels purposeful and pursue it wholeheartedly. It will set you on the path to happy retirement.

The Parent–Child Relationship in the Golden Years

Changing Roles

As we age, we realize that acceptance is critical to finding peace in the evening of life. Whether we are intent on worldly pursuits or have a more spiritual outlook, accepting the changes that come with aging can help us maintain our inner calm. It's natural to have a certain naivety in our younger years, believing that our children will always be there for us and never change. But as time passes, we understand that our children have their own lives and responsibilities. While we know they still care, we can't expect them to have as much time for us as they once did. By accepting this reality, we can free ourselves from unrealistic expectations and devote our time and energy to living our lives our way.

We are still part of a family, but it's worthwhile to remember that we are senior citizens, not first citizens. The children wish us well. They want us to have a good time, but our company is not as exciting anymore as it used to be when we were heroes to them and could do no wrong. Roles have changed. Now, they are heroes to their children. They find that role more exciting, and who can blame them?

We must accept these changing roles and priorities and define how we want to fit into the new equation. It would be best to do it ourselves rather than look to our children or others to lead us. Once we have accepted the new reality and decided how to live, new possibilities will open up. Now, we are untethered and free to chalk out our course of action independently. Being a parent and grandparent is lovely, and seeing your children grow up and have their children is fantastic. The roles may have shifted a bit, but love and connection remain. Embrace this new chapter of your life and enjoy every moment of it.

Parenting Doubts

If you're unsure about the job you did raising your children, please remember that children will not hold your parenting flaws against you. As they gain experience, children will recognize that you may have had flaws, but you did your best at the time. Instead, they will cherish the moments you spent together, the laughter and joy you shared. They are looking for memorable childhood moments to narrate to their children as stories. So don't harbour any remorse about what you should have done but failed to in raising your children. In the end, love counts above all. Be generous in expressing your love for your children. Appreciate and acknowledge their contribution to your life. Be genuine.

Family Problems

If you're struggling with family problems, such as sibling differences, matrimonial matters, divorce, etc., in your golden years, it's helpful to remember that your ability to influence the decisions of others is limited. Rather than sulking or complaining about not being consulted, it's best to practice silence and stay occupied with your routine, wearing a smile on your face. Try to see the positive side of the situation. Besides, staying out of controversial matters is better for our mental and physical health. Spend time with your friends, whether in person or online, and be happy and helpful. You've lived a long life and seen many challenges, but every generation faces its own difficulties. Wish your children well and give them your blessings—you'll leave behind happy memories.

Life After Loss of Spouse

The golden years can be especially challenging for someone left behind after losing their spouse. Even if the children are supportive, a surviving partner must navigate this stage of life alone (If they have chosen to remain single). When a couple has spent much of their life together, adjusting to life without their partner can be hard for the survivor. However, it's helpful to remember the wise words of the poet Maya Angelou: "Life will always go on, for it has no reason to stop, but it has reason to continue. No matter what happens, or how bad it seems today, life does go on, and it will be better tomorrow."

Those who are social and enjoy the company of others are more likely to find it easier to move on. Although they miss their partner, they do not become isolated after their passing.

Some spouses may discover new talents after their loss. With newfound time and independence, they may explore creative pursuits like writing, painting, or music, or find fulfillment in participating in community work. While it may be a challenging time, it's also an opportunity for personal growth and self-discovery.

Some individuals turn towards their spiritual beliefs for comfort and guidance. For those already part of a religious or spiritual community, this can be an opportunity to deepen their involvement and spend more time pursuing their spiritual aspirations, providing them with some solace and comfort.

Some struggle to overcome their regrets, and they dwell in the past. Sometimes, we might think about how we could have been a better partner, which can lead to isolation and guilt. But don't forget that we are not alone, and having a support system of family and friends can make all the difference. With the help of loved ones, we can begin to let go of the past and move forward with our lives.

> *"When you are sorrowful look again in your heart, and you shall see that in truth you are weeping for that which has been your delight."* —Kahlil Gibran

Everyone's healing journey is different, and finding a purpose that moves and inspires us can create new meaning in our lives. Being preoccupied with our grief is not the best way to heal and move forward.

Acts of kindness, no matter how small, can make a huge difference in transforming the way we feel about our loss. Simple gestures like visiting a friend or acquaintance in the hospital or at home—surprising them with a small gift, their favourite meal, or just chatting—can bring comfort and joy to both parties. It helps to view our loss from a broader perspective and feel empathy and compassion for our fellow beings.

Once we step out and get involved, we can find ways to contribute our skills, time, or resources to a cause that was dear to our departed partner or resonates with us. Even if we are home-bound, we can use our computer or cell phone to stay connected, and share our knowledge and experience to make a difference.

Here, I am reminded of my dear friend Shankar Mehta, a retired teacher, author, and counsellor who spent much time answering questions from the comfort of his home, helping people from all walks of life until the end.

Healing is a process, and finding a purpose can help us start a new chapter in our lives.

Reflections on the Golden Years of Life

The golden years of marriage are indeed a special time. It's a time to cherish the memories we've created and to make new ones with the people we love. Whether we choose to travel the world, pick up a new hobby, or enjoy the peace and quiet of our own home, the golden years are a period to live life to the fullest. It's also a time to express gratitude towards the people who have made it all possible, a time for acceptance, forgiveness, and spreading goodwill to all beings. These years are indeed an opportunity to count our blessings, and fill our minds and hearts with gratitude.

Looking back, I see that not everything happened how I wanted it to. At the micro level, quite a few things happened according to my plans. For example, I decided to migrate to Canada, and pursued it until I succeeded, although there were some constraints like age. But overall, I had not envisaged life as it has turned out to be. I came to Canada with two goals: to unite our family (to bring our two sons to Canada, who were studying/working in London, UK) and to build a successful business. Well, none of that happened. My sons are in Europe, nicely settled with their families, and my business was a non-starter, so I settled for less ambitious options.

Along the way, spirituality caught up with me. I had dabbled in it a few times before, but when I returned to it more intently, I was more earnest. Then, I started writing my motivational thoughts and essays and published my first book, *Inner Explorations of a Seeker*, in 2018. Now, I am writing my second book. I had not planned any of these developments. People go to India to seek spirituality. I reconnected with it in Canada!

When I write this, I am reminded of Steve Jobs' insightful words during his 2005 commencement speech at Stanford University: "You can't connect the dots looking forward; you can only connect them looking backwards. So, you have to trust that the dots will somehow connect in your future."

We must trust the journey.

Embracing the Joy of Slowing Down

The golden years of life are a time to savour and enjoy, to slow down and appreciate every activity, whether something as simple as eating, talking, shaving, applying makeup, taking a shower, or going for a walk. You don't have to rush to get anywhere—you've already arrived! You've worked hard and earned your wages, and now, every day is a bonus. Your priorities have shifted, and your parameters of efficiency and productivity are now different. So, take your time, relax, and enjoy life's beautiful moments.

My day begins with meditation and a leisurely sipping cup of tea. I try to share something inspirational daily—an insight, a thought, or a short essay. (I am devoting more time to completing this book now.) Having left behind an 8-to-5 work schedule, morning walks and afternoon naps are perks of the golden years I wouldn't bargain away for any other worldly gain. Writing and reading have replaced frequent parties, although I still enjoy participating in community events and getting together with like-minded people. I find shopping enjoyable, but I am not compulsive anymore. Gone are the days of rushing things; I savour solitude as much as companionship with my soulmate.

Slowing down can make every moment longer and our experience of living richer.

Balancing Financial Freedom and Peace of Mind

You're already doing better than most if you've reached financial independence. The goal should be to enjoy our golden years without the burden of financial stress, relying on a combination of work and state pensions or other sources of income. If we need to cut back on expenses to maintain a balanced budget, we should do so willingly and without hesitation. However, money doesn't equal happiness. Finding the peace we seek is hard if we are still caught up in the rat race. The secret to peace of mind, particularly in our golden years, is to be content and cultivate gratitude and forgiveness. That will make our golden years genuinely glorious.

Maintaining Health and Well-Being

As we age, our bodies undergo natural changes that can lead to physical challenges such as joint pain, decreased mobility, and chronic conditions. There are many steps we can take to maintain our health and well-being as we grow older. This includes staying active with regular exercise, eating a healthy diet, getting enough rest and sleep, and staying socially engaged with friends and family. It's also important to keep on top of medical screenings and check-ups and to work closely with healthcare providers to manage any chronic conditions or health concerns that may arise.

However, if we focus solely on the physical aspects of aging, we risk adopting a narrow perspective on life. Our physical and mental health are interconnected. Paying attention to our mental and spiritual well-being is as important as caring for our bodies. By incorporating meditation, yoga, reading, and listening to positive and spiritual material into our routines, we can develop a holistic outlook on life. The benefits of this balanced approach are immeasurable, offering a more enriched and fulfilling life.

Nonagenarian Krishan Bector, poet, scholar, and my esteemed friend summarizes his secret of a happy and healthy retired life: "Each day begins with a morning walk, a journey of two to four kilometres that renews the spirit. Age is just a number, never counted, never feared. Keeping a positive outlook and the company of fine, courteous and compassionate people, I try my best to live in the present. Love, the keystone that I seldom toss, remains the foundation of my life. I have an unswerving belief that exercise is the panacea to half of life's physical woes. Temperance in temper, I refuse to let hatred take root in me against anyone. At 90+, I am still active and live a purposeful life."

Embracing Change

Life is constantly evolving, and we must remain open to new experiences and perspectives. Our bodies naturally experience wear and tear and minor or major ailments as we age. Instead of worrying about these changes, we need to accept them as a part of the aging process and be prepared to handle them. Being realistic and accepting of these changes can help us reduce stress and look to the brighter side of aging.

Avoiding Stereotypes

Everyone has unique life experiences. Unfortunately, society tends to stereotype and label all older people as "elderly" without considering the diversity of their experiences and perspectives, and many seniors begin to internalize these misconceptions. Instead, we must recognize and celebrate the individuality of older individuals instead of just lumping them into one category.

We must balance our acceptance of natural changes as we age with a healthy skepticism of misconceptions around old age. For example, our reflections and movements slow down in later years, and we may take more time to perform tasks. But there is other side of the coin. With age comes the wisdom born of rich and varied experiences of life. It allows older people to see things from different angles and give more measured opinions and advice.

Also, later years are an opportunity to pursue the interests and passions we placed on the back burner because of work and family responsibilities. When we bring proper perspective to aging, this period can be one of opportunity and creativity rather than regret or loss.

Senator John Glenn, the oldest person to board a US Space Shuttle at age seventy-seven, exemplified the view that we shouldn't let age define us. In his memoir, he wisely said, "Too many people, when they get old, think that they have to live by the calendar. Letting ourselves be hemmed in by the chronological age may limit valuable opportunities."

I am a great fan of nonagenarian Dada Arjan Ajwani, a venerable community elder. At ninety-eight, he retains his phenomenal memory. Visitors are often surprised by how well he remembers pre-partition days (partition took place in India in 1947) and describes the names of places and people. He maintains close contact with his extended family and friends, particularly those needing guidance or company. (When I was writing this book, he used to call me to know how I was doing and inspired me to do my best.) Now, living in Coquitlam, BC, he is still in regular touch with the social and spiritual organizations he was part of in India.

I was curious to know the secret of his extraordinarily buoyant attitude and happy and healthy golden years, as I knew it would inspire others. So, I met him over tea to chat and ask questions. It's my pleasure to share the gist of our conversation with you.

QUESTION: Are you satisfied with how your life has turned out so far?

ANSWER: Yes, I am happy with how life has turned out. There have been ups and downs, but the spirit of adjustment has stood me well.

QUESTION: How do you spend your time?

ANSWER: I enjoy my time, listen to spiritual discourses, and don't interfere in my children's affairs. I let them live their lives as they want, according to their wishes. I only give them advice when asked.

QUESTION: Do you think retirement is a time to relax or pursue new interests and hobbies?

ANSWER: The world is changing so fast that your skills will become outdated by the time you retire. It is best to relax and enjoy your golden years rather than try to learn new skills.

QUESTION: How important are social connections in later years?

ANSWER: One should enjoy social gatherings and events but try to be happy without dependency on socializing.

QUESTION: What is your advice for people approaching retirement?

ANSWER: Try to enjoy life your way. Do not interfere in the affairs of your children. Don't offer unsolicited advice. Keep away from controversies. Having a spiritual anchor will help you be at peace with yourself, especially when experiencing the inevitable aches and pains of old age.

Living Lightly

The true value of life is found in living with ease and grace. This is particularly true in our later years. We cannot take material possessions with us when we leave this world, yet we continue accumulating things beyond our needs, nor will the people we are attached to accompany us, no matter how dear they are to us. Those who have already grasped this wisdom are truly blessed, but it's never too late to detach ourselves, as far as possible, from our possessions and people. It doesn't mean we should cut ourselves off from the world and become aloof or insensitive. We still love and treat people affectionately, enjoying things we like but with an attitude of detachment.

It's time to free ourselves of possessions we no longer need, unhealthy relationships that disempower us, and negative thoughts which rob us of optimism and aliveness. It will create more space for joy, peace, and contentment in our lives. Although it's not easy to break free from our old habits and ways of thinking, it's a gradual journey that begins with a change in our perspective.

"The beautiful journey of today can only begin when we learn to let go of yesterday." —Steve Maraboli

Liberating Power of Embracing Impermanence

"Impermanence is a principle of harmony. When we don't struggle against it, we are in harmony with reality." —Pema Chödrön

As we age and gain more life experience, we begin to understand the fleeting nature of life. It becomes easier to let go of things that once seemed so important and strive for the things that truly matter—peace of mind and purpose in our lives. While we have mixed emotions to acknowledge that our time on this earth is limited, it also brings a sense of clarity to our lives. We learn to appreciate each moment and cherish our time with loved ones. It's a poignant realization but one that ultimately brings peace and contentment.

Embracing the transient nature of life can free us from the fear of loss and anxiety of the future, allowing us to live more fully in the present.

Letting Go of Control and Enjoying the Anticipation

Have you ever considered stepping back and simply observing instead of actively participating? It may be difficult to relinquish control, but embracing this role during your golden years is rewarding. You are no longer a player, but that's perfectly fine. Rather than feeling compelled to do so, choose to enjoy being a spectator. It's no longer your responsibility, so try to step back and let things happen as they will. Imagine yourself sitting in a departure lounge, fully aware that anything could happen at any moment. It's time to wait and watch as life unfolds before you. And it will be helpful to remember the wise words of the ancient Chinese philosopher Confucius: "Old age, believe me, is a good and pleasant thing. It is true you are gently shouldered off the stage, but then you are given such a comfortable front stall as a spectator."

Prioritizing Our Partner

We experience greater physical and emotional interdependence with our partners as we age. We may find ourselves with children and grandchildren. While we should do what we can to help and support our children, our priority should always be our partner. It can be all too easy to neglect our significant other in favour of our children or sometimes even our social connections, but this can have sad consequences for our marriage.

Let our relationships remain full of substance and joy throughout our golden years, and let our emotional connections with our partner endure even as our passions cool with age.

"Making your relationship a top priority, even when you have kids, is truly a secret to a happy marriage." —Unknown

Finding Love in Later Years

A couple can find love for each other at any point in a marriage, even in the golden years, provided mutual respect between them is intact. When a couple has respect for one another, their love grows much deeper than just passion. After years of being together, they understand their spouse is their closest companion and confidant. If they don't take care of one another, then who will? With this realization, they become each other's priority, and their love naturally flourishes. They let go of the past and any complaints they may have had. Their relationship becomes harmonious, and they become closer than ever before. They communicate without blame and listen with patience and interest, and angry exchanges become a thing of the past. It is indeed a blissful life that is worth waiting for. This is possible when the couple practices restraint in their conduct and doesn't let mutual respect slip away. It will also be helpful to remember the wise words of author and physician Dr. Charles F. Glassman, also known as CoachMD: "Love is not always fireworks and magic. Often, we'll experience it in the form of patience, acceptance, loyalty, and mutual respect."

Discovering Hidden Talents

Retirement can be an opportunity to discover hidden talents. After spending a lifetime pursuing our careers, retirement may sound like a daunting prospect. However, once we overcome our initial fears, we may discover talents we never knew we had. With busy work and family life as priorities, we may not have explored our passions fully. Now, with new freedom and the luxury of time, we can turn our attention to matters dear to our hearts. That can include travel, spiritual pursuits, hobbies, community, social groups, spending time with family, or pursuing hidden talents.

It's never too late to discover new talents and pursue our passions.

Spirit of Giving

Our family, community, country, and the universe have given us so much, and it's time to give back. Everything we do now should have a touch of giving. Pursue this with urgency, as time is limited. By thinking about how we can help others and ease their pain and suffering, we not only positively impact their lives but also find meaning and fulfillment in our own lives. It's a win–win situation, and it's something we can do every day in interactions with those around us.

Surendra Handa and Sanyogita Handa, from Surrey, BC, are an inspiring example. Despite their senior years and health challenges, they remain passionately engaged in community service. They organize activities like yoga, bingo, and summer picnics for seniors, and even arrange talks by health experts to provide helpful advice to seniors.

They do all of this with a smile and treat everyone with respect. Their positive attitude uplifts and inspires others and helps them cope with their ailments. When we focus on others, we have less time to worry about our own problems.

"Giving back to society and community enriches our lives, making it a double blessing." —*Kellie Sullivan*

Be a Storyteller

As we age, we often find ourselves reminiscing about our lives and the experiences we've had. It's natural to feel like we can't keep up with the younger generations, and we don't have to. This is the time to relax and take it easy. However, if you want something to do, why not become a storyteller? With all your experiences, you have a wealth of stories to share that can inspire, motivate, entertain, and amuse others. Your grandchildren and younger generations will especially love hearing these stories. Share your wisdom and the lessons you've learned along the way. You might even learn something from them in return.

And the best part? You don't need to be an erudite or well-read person to be a storyteller. You'll be amazed to find kids love to listen to the same stories and enjoy them time and time again. I remember sitting around my grandmother after dinner, listening to her stories. We remembered every detail of the stories she shared with us and loved every minute of it. Before beginning the story, she would ask us which story we wanted to listen to that night. We would say the story of the lion or prince and snake and enjoy it as if we were hearing it for the first time.

We often hear that kids these days are smart and know more than us. While this may be true when it comes to technology, there is no substitute for experience. Grandparents have much to offer their grandchildren, and sharing a piece of your experience or wisdom can prove invaluable to them. So, seize every opportunity to share your stories and knowledge with the younger generations. You never know how it may help them on their journeys through life.

Aging Gracefully

If we can accept and embrace our age, we can truly enjoy our later years and all the experiences that come with each passing year. Getting older is a privilege that not everyone gets to experience, so we should do our best to make the most of it and value every moment.

While it can be tempting to cling to the passions of youth, remember that decay is a natural part of the process. Instead of dwelling on what we've lost, let's make the most of the time we have left.

Let's spread joy to those around us and find happiness in the company of loved ones, friends, and even strangers.

Treating people with love and kindness drives away emptiness and brings fullness to our lives. Constantly complaining or trying to manipulate and guilt-trip our loved ones can only lead to resentment and distance. On the other hand, they are touched and moved when we communicate our needs and concerns in a respectful and dignified manner, show our appreciation, and acknowledge their contribution to our lives.

When we approach aging with grace and gratitude, our golden years can be some of the best years of our lives.

"To age with grace is to paint life's canvas with strokes of wisdom and hues of experience." —Unknown

Staying Relevant in Later Years

As we enter our golden years, our relevance is not determined by others but by how we treat ourselves. Creating conditions supporting our independence is necessary to maintain a belief in ourselves. Living independently, as long as possible, allows us to choose our daily routines, plan our vacations, and stay connected with the people we love. By taking control of our lives, we can avoid feeling irrelevant and continue to thrive in our golden years.

Also, finding a purpose that inspires us to make a difference can help us stay relevant at any age. And it doesn't have to be significant. For example, I know a few retired people who regularly call or visit members of their community who are alone to cheer them up or offer help. It's their way of making a difference in the world.

Making the Most of Our Golden Years

Happiness is a personal journey, and every journey is unique. While our family and friends can provide love and support, ultimately, it's up to us to find joy and fulfillment in life.

The things that brought us happiness in the past may not work anymore, so we must explore new avenues to find our joy. For example, if money and success were the driving forces of our lives, they may not be sufficient to give us peace and contentment in the later years. We need to look deeper into our experiences to see what makes us come alive and fills us with hope. The key is to pursue what resonates with us. Joy and contentment will naturally flow once we have discovered something that gives meaning to our lives.

In his early eighties, Mohan Bhojwani is truly blessed with a caring wife, Rani, and a family. He has a passion for music and writing and an attitude of acceptance and gratitude, but unfortunately, he suffers from chronic back pain. Despite this, Mohan remains positive and makes the most of his situation. He even jokes about his back pain, saying it's been with him for so long it doesn't want to part with him. Mohan practices yoga and goes to a chiropractor but never complains about his condition. He accepts it and does what he can to manage it. Mohan's positive attitude is truly inspiring and a testament to his resilience.

Beauty of Solitude

It's a blessing to enjoy solitude. It helps avoid falling prey to boredom and loneliness in later years.

"I have never found a companion that was so companionable as solitude." —Henry David Thoreau

We never know when it's time for us to leave this world, and it's unlikely that both partners will depart at the same time. While we may be fortunate enough to have a supportive network of loved ones, the bond built over the years is irreplaceable.

We'll still have friends and family to enjoy their company, but we'll also appreciate the time we spend alone.

Cherishing Memories

The golden years of our lives are filled with many memories we can cherish forever. Playing hide-and-seek and doing crazy things we never thought possible. Our first crush, perhaps on the teacher, our first romance, and our first date. How we couldn't wait to grow up and be free to do things our way without having to ask for permission all the time. Our sporting days, wild parties, and drunken brawls. Our acts of kindness and service. Our graduation ceremonies and the proud looks of our parents. All of these memories are priceless and will stay with us forever.

> *"The best things in life are the people you love, the places you have seen, and the memories you have made along the way."* —Unknown

Embracing Self-Acceptance

As we get older, we realize that it's not necessary to constantly try to change people's perceptions of us. We have reached a point where we are secure in our self-knowledge and know who we are. We have the patience to let people discover who we are at their own pace, and if they never do, that's okay, too. At the end of the day, what matters most is how comfortable we are in our own skin.

> *"The closing years of life are like the end of a masquerade party, when the masks are dropped."* —Arthur Schopenhauer

We have a chance to break free from the expectations of others and embrace our true selves. The pressures of family, work, and society we faced in our active years no longer apply. We can be ourselves without worrying about pleasing others. Those around us will accept us, maybe explaining away our quirks of old age. Don't consider this as a condescending attitude. These are the perks of old age.

We tend to explain and justify our every decision, but with experience, we realize it's not worth the energy. When disagreements or arguments arise, it's best to practice dignified silence and let them pass. It's a peaceful and respectful way to handle unpleasant encounters, particularly in our later years.

It's not suggested we become self-centered, complaining, fault-finding seniors in our golden years. No, not at all. It's an opportunity to be yourself and spend your time your way without hurting others. Your family, friends and society may still expect you to conform to certain stereotypes. Let's give them a polite nod and continue the last stage of the journey in our own way.

Embracing Imperfection

The older I get, the more amazed I am at how often I make mistakes and how frequently my assumptions turn out to be wrong. Age may bring experience, but it doesn't make us immune to errors. We all have the potential to be wrong and to learn from our mistakes. Some people pretend they have all the answers and never ask questions, while others are more open-minded and willing to listen and learn. Being vulnerable and acknowledging our mistakes rather than pretending to be perfect is liberating. Changing our minds based on new information shows maturity and growth, not weakness.

> *"There is beauty and humility in imperfection." —Guillermo del Toro*

By embracing imperfection, we can avoid stress and be more relaxed, as we don't have to set unrealistic standards for ourselves. Besides, we will be less eager to judge others, knowing we all are on the same boat. It will make us more accepting of ourselves and others, radiating warmth and compassion.

Kindness Always Matters

Besides being a noble habit, treating people with kindness and respect is rewarding. We feel good, as being kind expresses our basic nature as human beings and brings sunshine to other people's lives.

I have known Mark for fifteen years. He is now in his early nineties. He became a widower when he was in his late eighties. He lives independently and has all the ailments a person his age is expected to have. But that doesn't stop him from enjoying life. He still drives, relishes good food, and regularly goes out with his friends. He keeps his doctors in good humour; they look after him well.

He keeps in touch with his community; they visit him when he is not well or in the hospital. He asks them to prepare dishes of his choice, and they do, and they happily deliver them to him. I have often wondered how he can connect with people so well despite living life on his terms. And the answer that comes to my mind is that he is kind and respectful to people in his daily life.

It is heartwarming to see how Mark has built such strong community connections. He exemplifies how being kind and respectful can go a long way in building meaningful relationships. In a world where we often get caught up in our lives, it is worth remembering the value of kindness and how it can positively impact those around. Moreover, as the Ancient Greek storyteller wisely said, "No act of kindness, no matter how small, is ever wasted."

Navigating Life's Surprises

"Life is full of surprises. Not all of these are pleasant, so you need to be ready for what life brings you." —Unknown

Unexpected changes or surprises shape our relationships and reveal the true strength of our bonds. Partners who face life's surprises with love, resilience, and compassion create enduring stories worth celebrating.

A Life Well-Lived

Sometimes, we may face health challenges that can turn our lives upside down. A diagnosis of a disease like cancer can be challenging to cope with. It can drastically alter our lifestyle and leave us feeling lost and overwhelmed.

A dear friend of mine was diagnosed with cancer recently. Despite the devastating news, she remained calm and serene. She says, "I am in the evening of my life. I have lived my life to the fullest. It has been a wonderful journey with all its ups and downs and precious memories. God is always with me. I have faith in my master's teachings. Watching him and listening to his discourses gives me the strength to face any situation. Besides, I am grateful to have the support of caring family and friends. I have no complaints. I am ready for whatever has to happen."

Her positive outlook and acceptance of the situation are truly inspiring. She was not giving in to self-pity or asking, "Why me?" Instead, she was determined to pursue whatever treatment options were available with strength and grace. Seeing her peaceful demeanour and positive perspective on life, even under challenging conditions, has left a lasting impact on me. It's a reminder that even in the toughest of times, we can find inner peace and strength through spirituality.

What I Know Now

In conclusion, our golden years are a period to nourish our bodies and souls. It's time to practice gratitude and forgiveness and let go of any lingering regrets, remorse, or resentments against ourselves or others.

As we enter our golden years, let's recognize the transitory nature of our existence on this earth. This is a time to practice detachment, to be content with what we have, and to value the present moment.

As the evening of our lives approaches, it's time to ignite the lamp within, to illuminate our inner space with peace and the wisdom that comes with age, and remember that we are all in the same boat and need a fair dose of generosity to make our and others' journeys on this earth pleasant.

Afterword

This book would only be complete if I shared the experiences of our own life journeys. When I asked Komal, my wife, whether she would like to share her feelings and thoughts about our life journey, she came up with an honest, straightforward, and warm account. It's my pleasure to share it here.

> I was born and brought up in India. We have completed fifty-two years of marriage. Times have changed. It was different back then; now, it's different, but life is the same. It was good then, and now also it's going well. When there is mutual respect and care, love finds its place. If we focus on negative experiences, the positive experiences will get sidetracked. When we try to see the positive side of a relationship and appreciate each other, our life experiences will be different.
>
> Communication is important. But more important is making major life

decisions together, which we always did, whether it was moving houses, selecting a school for our children, planning vacations, watching movies, buying household goods, or anything else.

It's natural to have differences of opinion and outlook. However, if there is honesty in the relationship, it's easy to understand one another. We must listen to each other, and for that, we need patience. We did not make a big deal of our differences and did not blow small things out of proportion. If there were any flare-ups, we let things cool down.

Then, children grew up and settled down, grandchildren came, and our lives became more joyful. Amar and I live together and passionately pursue our hobbies and interests. Amar has a passion for writing and meditation. I love gardening and writing poems in my simple language. We look after each other and our health. We have a circle of lovely friends.

Despite the ups and downs of life's journey, I feel a deep sense of gratitude for everything and everyone in my life and for the Almighty. I feel complete.

I couldn't have said it better. Our relationship has acquired depth and maturity, just like a mature tree whose roots have gone deeper, faced the rough and fair weather, and stood the test of time. Do we still have differences and disagreements? You bet. But they are like lines on the water. You put a finger in the water, which will stir the water for a moment, but the water will return to its earlier shape in no time.

I can't think of life without Komal. Of course, we both know one of us must traverse the last passage of our journey on our own. And, we are ready: She with her gardening and poems, I with my writing and meditation, with a river of precious memories flowing that death cannot erase. We have a lot to be grateful for in the blessings of life.

And so do all of us.

Life Principles

1. Spirituality is a beautiful companion. It makes the end of the earthly journey peaceful.
2. Love people, but love yourself first. Self-compassion is the gateway to compassion for all.
3. Cultivate equanimity. It's the anchor for life's rough weather.
4. Make peace of mind your priority. Avoid saying and doing things you may regret later.
5. Money is not everything, but financial freedom is necessary to live with a free mind.
6. Look after yourself. The body is a valuable tool for living well and doing well.
7. Let people learn from you, but don't waste time on those who cannot appreciate your value. Wish them well and move on.
8. Do what needs to be done, but with a state of detachment. You don't have to prove yourself.
9. As far as possible, be independent, but not aloof.
10. Surround yourself with positive and supportive people who uplift and inspire you.
11. Spend some time with nature. It never rejects.

12. Cultivate a positive mindset and practice gratitude daily.
13. Practice forgiveness. In addition to being a noble virtue, forgiveness reduces stress in our lives.
14. To live life to the fullest, learn to enjoy life in the slow lane.
15. Be humble. Arrogance is self-defeating.
16. Better choices translate into a better life. Trust the journey.
17. Pursue hobbies and interests that bring you joy and fulfillment.
18. It's time to step back and let others take the lead.
19. Solitude sings the sweetest song. When we learn to enjoy our own company, we are never bored.
20. Never give up on yourself. The game is over when we do.

Acknowledgements

I have met some extraordinary people and learned so much from them on my life journey. I thank each one of them. Their wisdom, compassion, and kindness continue to inspire me.

I sincerely appreciate and thank the following people for their wholehearted help in the making of this book:

Pradeep Atrey, notable author and my friend, for providing valuable suggestions. His genuine kindness and spontaneous support, without much ado, are disarming.

Terence Morris, PhD, has been my friend for many years. He painstakingly reviewed the manuscript and gave helpful feedback. His support over the years has given me much strength.

Krishan Bector, a poet and scholar, and my esteemed friend, for his unwavering belief in my work and heartwarming kindness.

Thank you to Surendra Handa and Sanyogita Handa for allowing me to share their work. Their community service and endearing nature inspire many of us.

Mohan Bhojwani, my friend, for sharing his life experience. He inspires many of us with his positive thoughts and soulful music.

I want to pay tribute to my late friend, author, and educator, Shankar Mehta. His warm and generous appreciation of my work and our occasional Thursday luncheon meetings are memories I will always cherish.

I especially thank Dada Arjan Ajwani for the lively chat (which is included in this book) and his kind blessings.

A big thank you to Dinah Laprairie, my editor, for helping me take this book to a new level. Her meticulous approach and attention to detail motivated me to make it as complete a guide on marriage and retirement as possible.

With all its ups and downs, spending fifty-two years with my wife has been my life's blessing and love. As always, she has provided unconditional support and indispensable feedback. Her contribution to making this book happen is as much as mine.